How To Boost
Metabolism With Food

How To Boost Metabolism With Food

The Ray Peat Diet
for Thyroid Health and Fast
Metabolism

Benedicte Mai Lerche MSc PhD
BiochemNordic

"Healing Metabolism"

Book 3

ISBN: 978-87-975361-0-0 (Paperback)

ISBN: 978-87-975361-1-7 (Hardcover)

ISBN: 978-87-975361-2-4 (E-book)

A note to the reader:

The author of this book shares research from Dr. Ray Peat and other sources, which may be considered controversial and subject to varying opinions among experts. The content of this book, including but not limited to text, graphics, images, tables, and other material, is offered for informational purposes only and is not intended to replace professional medical advice, diagnosis, or treatment. Readers are strongly encouraged to consult with their physician or another qualified health provider for any questions related to a medical condition or health concerns. Neither the author nor the publisher makes any express or implied representations or warranties concerning the information's suitability, reliability, timeliness, or accuracy. The author and publisher are not responsible for any consequences resulting from the use or misuse of the information in this book. They specifically disclaim any liability for personal or other loss, risk, or harm that may be incurred, directly or indirectly, as a result of using or applying any content of this book. Readers should be aware that applying this information to their lives is a personal decision and responsibility.

Book Series

Through my "Healing Metabolism" book series, I am dedicated to sharing Dr. Ray Peat's health research. The series aims to deepen readers' understanding and offer practical methods for overcoming metabolic and hormonal imbalances, utilizing diet, thyroid replacement therapy, hormonal support compounds, and other lifestyle changes.

Book 1:

The first book, "How I Overcame Hypothyroidism," chronicles my personal health journey and victory over low thyroid function (hypothyroidism) using Dr. Ray Peat's health approach. It introduces Dr. Peat's research and equips readers with a fundamental understanding of his key health concepts for healing metabolism.

Book 2:

The second book, "Test Your Thyroid Function," delves into Dr. Ray Peat's principles for thyroid testing and the diagnosis of hypothyroidism. This volume provides crucial knowledge for understanding thyroid blood tests and explains how to use pulse rate and body temperature to track your metabolism at home. Additionally, it covers essential aspects of thyroid function and metabolic health.

Book 3:

The current book explores Dr. Ray Peat's nutritional research, offering a detailed and approachable explanation of his pro-metabolic diet principles.

Future volumes:

I am developing further volumes for the "Healing Metabolism" series. Upcoming books will provide insights into topics such as thyroid medication and hormonal support supplements like progesterone and pregnenolone.

Support my work:

If you find any of my books helpful, I would be extremely grateful if you could take a few minutes to leave a short review on the platform where you purchased the book or on Goodreads. This will help other potential readers dealing with similar health issues discover and benefit from my work.

Contents

Dedication

With deep appreciation, this book is dedicated to the late Dr. Ray Peat, whose exceptional health research and generous support have restored the metabolic health of many, including my own.

Raymond Franklin Peat (1936-2022), a distinguished American researcher with a Ph.D. in biology, devoted over five decades to studying the interactions of nutrition, hormones, and health. His pioneering work on diet, thyroid function, progesterone, pregnenolone, and related hormones has left an indelible impact on these fields and positively influenced the lives of numerous individuals struggling with metabolic health issues.

In my early twenties, I suffered from hypothyroidism, a severe form of slow metabolism that caused a range of symptoms including chronic fatigue, severe digestive issues, muscle pain, headaches, low blood sugar, eczema, allergies, and hormonal imbalances among others. Fortunately, my encounter with Dr. Ray Peat marked the turning point in my struggle with this condition.

Learning about his work gave me the essential roadmap I needed to restore my metabolic function. Dr. Ray Peat introduced me to his unique treatment protocol, which included diet adjustments, the right thyroid medication, and hormonal support supplements like progesterone and pregnenolone.

Inspired by my recovery, I pursued a degree in biochemistry at university and later established my website, biochemnordic.com. Through my website and books, I now share Dr. Ray Peat's health principles.

In this book, I will explore the pro-metabolic dietary principles I learned from Dr. Peat, highlighting their role in boosting the metabolic rate and improving thyroid health.

Dr. Ray Peat's dietary principles are not merely a quick fix but a comprehensive nutritional lifestyle. By learning how to support your metabolism with the right foods, you can reduce stress, inflammation, aging, and disease.

My goal with this book is to cover all significant aspects of Dr. Peat's nutritional research, presenting a flexible and practical diet that avoids fanaticism and rigidity. This approach will help you easily integrate his nutritional advice into your daily routines.

It's important to note that this book reflects my interpretation of Dr. Peat's dietary approach. Others may apply his principles slightly differently than what is presented here.

I hope this book acts as a beacon for those navigating the complex world of health and nutrition, enabling them to embark on their journey toward metabolic healing using Dr. Ray Peat's dietary principles.

Benedicte Mai Lerche, MSc, PhD

August 2024

Benedicte Mai Lerche MSc PhD

Introduction

The metabolic rate quantifies how swiftly we transform food into energy. Many people link a slow metabolic rate with weight gain and obesity; however, it's critical to recognize that a very slow metabolism is a serious health condition known as hypothyroidism (Barnes & Galton, 1976, pp. 17-25).

As your metabolism decreases, each cell in your body generates less energy. In this low-energy state, the body loses structure and control, which can allow harmful degenerative processes to unfold (Peat R., Generative Energy, 2001a, pp. 1-5).

While a slow metabolism often results in weight gain, it can also lead to more serious health issues, such as chronic fatigue, digestive problems, hair and skin issues, hormonal imbalances as well as stress, inflammation, premature aging, and much more (Barnes & Galton, 1976, pp. 20-25).

The dietary principles outlined in this book are tailored for anyone seeking to enhance their metabolic rate through a scientifically supported dietary approach.

The diet advice presented in this book is drawn from Dr. Peat's distinctive nutritional research, which spanned over five decades.

Dr. Peat's nutritional principles are designed to shift the body into a higher metabolic state, fostering repair, healing, and vibrant health.

He emphasized that many traditional and health-focused diets often contain foods that directly suppress the metabolic rate.

Upon my initial interaction with Dr. Ray Peat, he advised me to avoid many foods commonly regarded as healthy such as polyunsaturated fats, beans, lentils, nuts, seeds, soy products, and raw vegetables from the cabbage family (Peat R., Generative Energy, 2001a, p. 75; Peat R., Nutrition for Women: 100 Short Articles, 2001d, p. 17).

The nutritional landscape is fraught with misconceptions that lack a solid basis in true biochemistry.

Frequent claims such as "sugar is poison," "milk is only for children," and "saturated fats cause heart disease," are often made without a scientifically sound explanation of how these foods impact the health of the body.

It is important to note that this book is not a cookbook; rather, its goal is to dispel many misconceptions about diet and demonstrate how adhering to Dr. Ray Peat's nutritional guidelines can boost your metabolism.

Since Dr. Ray Peat's dietary guidelines differ significantly from other advice, I will thoroughly elucidate the rationale behind each of his dietary recommendations.

Prepare yourself for a book that will fundamentally challenge everything you thought you knew about diet and health.

By the end of this book, you should be equipped to eliminate foods from your diet that inhibit your metabolism and instead base your meals on pro-metabolic combinations of the right types of food.

Although Dr. Peat has not detailed a specific diet plan, his nutritional recommendations have evolved over the years, and currently, those who adhere to his principles refer to it as the "Ray Peat diet."

Before exploring these dietary principles, it's crucial to discuss key aspects of metabolism, which is the focus of the first chapter of this book.

The book is structured as follows:

Chapter 1: This chapter delves into essential aspects of metabolism, detailing the function of the thyroid gland and how the active thyroid hormone controls your metabolic rate. You'll learn about common symptoms of a sluggish metabolism, the best methods for testing your metabolic rate, and the causes and triggers of hypothyroidism.

Chapter 2: In this crucial chapter, I examine why polyunsaturated fats, often touted as healthy, actually pose significant risks to your health and thyroid function. You'll discover how these fats became mislabeled as healthy, their role in severely suppressing metabolism, and their contribution to obesity. Additionally, I discuss the benefits of saturated fats, which improve health and enhance metabolic function.

Chapter 3: This chapter explains how maintaining stable blood sugar amplifies the metabolic rate and examines the varied impacts of different carbohydrates on blood sugar and digestion. As you progress through this chapter, your perception of sugars, fruits, starches, whole grains, and fiber will transform. Ultimately, you'll gain profound insights into which carbohydrates boost metabolism and which ones predispose you to obesity.

Chapter 4: This chapter emphasizes the importance of consuming high-quality protein every day. You'll learn why many plant-based and some animal-based proteins can harm your health and hinder metabolic function. Additionally, you'll discover why excessive meat consumption may not be suitable for adults. By the end of this chapter, you will be able to select the best types of protein for optimal liver and metabolic function.

Chapter 5: In this chapter, I explore why consuming sufficient salt is particularly important for people with a slow metabolic rate. You'll discover how salt prevents water retention and high blood pressure, contrary to popular misconceptions. I also explain the types of salt and spices that align with the principles of the "Ray Peat diet."

Chapter 6: This chapter focuses on beverages, explaining why excessive water intake can be detrimental to your health. It discusses the benefits of caffeine, the consumption of coffee and tea, and which types of alcoholic drinks are acceptable.

Chapter 7: This chapter explores food additives, emphasizing their role as contributors to inflammation and disease. You'll gain insight into various common food additives and understand how they harm your body.

Chapter 8: This chapter summarizes key points about fats, carbohydrates, and protein, guiding you in combining foods optimally for stable blood sugar and a higher metabolic rate. You'll learn why frequent eating and a bedtime meal can lower stress and improve sleep.

Chapter 9: The final chapter goes beyond diet, outlining other aspects of Dr. Ray Peat's health philosophy for healing metabolism, including thyroid replacement therapy, hormonal support compounds, nutritional supplements, light therapy, and more.

Chapter 1: Metabolism

Benedicte Mai Lerche MSc PhD

What is Metabolism

To fully understand Dr. Ray Peat's pro-metabolic diet, it's essential to first grasp the key facets of metabolism. This chapter is dedicated specifically to that purpose.

Metabolism involves all the chemical reactions within the body's cells that convert food into biological energy. This biological energy then powers essential cellular functions and reactions (Nava & Raja., 2022).

Chemically, metabolism refers to the process in which cells use oxygen (O_2) to transform nutrients (food) into carbon dioxide (CO_2), water (H_2O), heat, and adenosine triphosphate (ATP). ATP serves as the body's biological energy source (Barnes & Galton, 1976, p. 3; Vander, Sherman, & Luciano, 2001, pp. 619-620).

To exemplify, consider the metabolic process involving glucose, represented by the following equation (Vander, Sherman, & Luciano, 2001, pp. 619-620; Boston University School of Public Health, 2017):

$$C_6H_{12}O_6 + 6O_2 \rightarrow 6CO_2 + 6H_2O + Heat + ATP$$

The speed of metabolism, or the metabolic rate, determines how quickly the body converts food into energy. Individuals with a high metabolism burn a substantial number of calories, and their cells produce a significant amount of biological energy (ATP) (Barnes & Galton, 1976, pp. 18-19).

While many associate the metabolic rate primarily with weight management, Dr. Ray Peat emphasized that a high metabolic rate is essential for maintaining good health. He explained the critical importance of biological energy (ATP) for maintaining the structure and function of the body's tissues and organs (Peat R., Generative Energy, 2001a, pp. 1-5).

Dr. Peat proposed that disease, inflammation, and degeneration arise when there's an imbalance between the body's energy production and the demands of its environment (Peat R., Generative Energy, 2001a, pp. 1-5).

This indicates that a slow metabolic rate, marked by low cellular energy levels, significantly contributes to the onset of harmful degenerative processes (Peat R., Nutrition for Women: 100 Short Articles, 2001d, p. 16).

The thyroid gland plays a pivotal role in regulating the speed of metabolism. Therefore, a reduced metabolic rate can also be termed low thyroid function, medically known as hypothyroidism.

In the following section, I will delve into crucial aspects of thyroid function and its relationship to metabolism.

Benedicte Mai Lerche MSc PhD

Thyroid & Metabolism

Located in the front of the throat, the human thyroid gland (Figure 1.1) has a butterfly shape (Barnes & Galton, 1976, p. 3).

It is a small endocrine gland that produces and releases two hormones: triiodothyronine (T3), and thyroxine (T4) into the bloodstream. Collectively, T4 and T3 are known as the thyroid hormones (Society of Endocrinology, 2020).

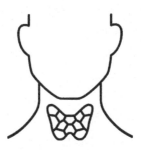

Figure 1.1: A sketch of the human thyroid gland, illustrating its distinctive butterfly shape and its location at the front of the throat.

It is crucial to understand that T3 is the active thyroid hormone, which affects cells and regulates the metabolic rate, whereas T4 is a pro-hormone for T3 (Society of Endocrinology, 2020).

The thyroid gland secretes more T4 than T3 (American Thyroid Association, 2023a). Dr. Peat, explained that T4 and T3 are released in a ratio of about 3:1, which corresponds to 75% T4 and 25% T3 (Peat R., Generative Energy, 2001a, p. 73).

Once secreted by the thyroid gland, T4 can be converted to the active thyroid hormone T3 in other organs and tissues (Society of Endocrinology, 2020).

Most of this conversion occurs in the liver, which allows the liver to regulate the production of the active thyroid hormone T3 (Peat R., Generative Energy, 2001a, p. 73).

Because T3 regulates the speed of the metabolic rate that converts food into energy, T3 essentially controls the body's energy (ATP) supply (Vander, Sherman, & Luciano, 2001, p. 267).

Hypothyroidism, characterized by low T3 levels, has devastating effects on the body, leading to various symptoms. This occurs because low cellular energy prevents tissues and organs from functioning optimally. In the following section, I will list the common symptoms associated with hypothyroidism.

> **Key Points – Metabolism & Thyroid Function:**
>
> The metabolic rate measures how quickly food is converted into biological energy (ATP).
>
> The active thyroid hormone T3 controls the speed of metabolism.
>
> A slow metabolic rate can also be referred to as low thyroid function or hypothyroidism.

Benedicte Mai Lerche MSc PhD

Symptoms of Slow Metabolism

A slow metabolic rate means that each cell in your body produces little energy. In a state of reduced metabolism, the body is more prone to harmful and degenerative processes rather than repair and healing (Peat R., Nutrition for Women: 100 Short Articles, 2001d, p. 16).

A slow metabolism affects various bodily functions including energy levels, temperature regulation, heart rate, and overall hormonal health. Low T3 also affects organs such as the adrenals, pancreas, and reproductive glands (Barnes & Galton, 1976, p. 20). Therefore, a slow metabolic rate is significant not only for weight management but also for overall health.

The condition of slow metabolism, also known as low thyroid function or hypothyroidism, may affect various body systems, although not necessarily to the same extent in every individual. Therefore, the symptoms of slow metabolism can vary from person to person (Barnes & Galton, 1976, pp. 22-25).

Below is a list of common symptoms associated with a slow metabolic rate (Barnes & Galton, 1976, pp. 22-24; Wilson, 2015, p. 25; Peat R., Nutrition for

Women: 100 Short Articles, 2001d, pp. 16-18; Peat R., From PMS to Menopause: Female Hormones in Context, 2001b, p. 78).

Common low metabolic symptoms:

This list, while not exhaustive, provides an overview of the diverse symptoms related to slow metabolism (low thyroid function). It's important to remember that not all symptoms need to be present for you to have a metabolic problem.

Fatigue: Feeling tired and lacking energy, even after getting adequate rest (chronic fatigue).

Headaches: Experiencing pressure headaches and migraines.

Hypoglycemia: Having low blood sugar, resulting in a need to eat frequently to avoid feeling faint and dizzy.

Weight changes: Experiencing unexplained weight gain or difficulty losing weight despite maintaining a healthy diet and regular exercise routine. Some individuals may also experience weight loss.

Low body temperature: Having cold intolerance, feeling excessively cold even in warm temperatures, and having cold hands and feet.

Reduced heart rate: Experiencing a slow heart rate (bradycardia) and decreased heart function.

Heart problems & disease: Experiencing heart pain, poor heart sounds, enlargement of the heart, palpitations, and hypertension.

Constipation: Experiencing slow digestion, difficulty passing stools, and infrequent bowel movements.

Digestive problems: Painful digestion, irritable bowel syndrome (IBS), as well as an overgrowth of bad bacteria and candida.

Dry skin: Having dry, rough, thin, pale skin that may be itchy and scaly, accompanied by conditions like eczema or skin infections.

Brittle hair & nails: Experiencing thinning of hair and nails, hair loss, changes in hair texture, and potential loss of the outer third of the eyebrows.

Muscle and joint pain: Experiencing muscle aches, stiffness, and joint pain not attributed to any specific injury or physical activity.

Carpal tunnel syndrome: Having pain, numbness, and tingling sensations in the hand, arms, and fingers (carpal tunnel syndrome).

Mood changes: Experiencing depression, anxiety, irritability, and mood swings.

Cognitive impairment: Having difficulty concentrating, poor memory, and decreased mental alertness (brain fog).

Hoarseness: Experiencing a deepening or hoarse voice, often accompanied by a sore throat.

Swelling: Experiencing water retention (edema), often with swelling or puffiness in the face, hands, feet, or ankles.

High cholesterol: Having elevated levels of cholesterol in the blood, even with a healthy diet and lifestyle.

Decreased libido: Experiencing a loss of interest in sexual activity and a reduced sexual drive.

Menstrual irregularities: Having irregular menstrual cycles, heavy menstrual bleeding, prolonged menstrual periods, painful menstruation, and experiencing symptoms of premenstrual syndrome (PMS) and polycystic ovaries (PCOS).

Infertility & miscarriage: Experiencing male and female infertility, with a higher chance of miscarriage in females.

Insomnia: Having problems falling asleep and/or waking up during the night.

Other symptoms: Poor vision, hearing loss, anemia, allergies, frequent colds, infections, orange calluses, inflammation, premature aging, and more.

Benedicte Mai Lerche MSc PhD

Measure Your Metabolism

To assess a patient's metabolic rate, doctors often perform blood tests to evaluate thyroid function, typically measuring levels of TSH (Thyroid Stimulating Hormone), T4 (thyroxine), and T3 (triiodothyronine). Other crucial tests include those for reverse T3 and thyroid antibodies.

You may have already undergone some of these tests and found your results to be within the so-called "normal" ranges.

It's crucial to understand that you can still have a low metabolism despite normal thyroid blood test results.

One reason is that the reference ranges for these blood tests are quite broad, allowing many individuals with symptoms of hypothyroidism to fall within these "normal" ranges. Dr. Ray Peat explained the importance of distinguishing between the normal reference ranges for thyroid blood tests and the optimal levels for these tests, which are more indicative of true thyroid health.

Additionally, Dr. Ray Peat pointed out that blood tests may not accurately reflect the true metabolic rate, as the cellular response to the active thyroid hormone T3 can be inhibited by anti-metabolic substances like polyunsaturated fats (Peat R., Generative Energy, 2001a, p. 72; Wilson, 2015, p. 28; Peat R., TSH, temperature, pulse rate, and other indicators in hypothyroidism, 2008a).

Dr. Peat recommended using a combination of thyroid function blood tests, pulse rate, and body temperature tracking, along with symptom monitoring, to more accurately gauge your metabolic rate.

Optimal metabolism is characterized by an oral temperature of approximately 98.6°F (37°C) and a pulse rate ranging from 80 to 85 beats per minute (Peat, 2001b, p. 76). (Peat, 2001b, p. 76).

It's essential to recognize that individuals with reduced thyroid function may compensate for their energy deficiency by producing high levels of stress hormones, such as cortisol and adrenaline. These hormones can elevate body temperature and pulse rate, potentially complicating the use of these metrics in evaluating the metabolic rate. (Peat, 2008, p. 5).

In my book, "Test Your Thyroid Function," you will discover essential information to help you interpret your thyroid blood test results and monitor your metabolism at home using pulse rate and body temperature. This book also explores many important aspects of metabolic health, including the autoimmune form of hypothyroidism known as Hashimoto's thyroiditis, reverse T3, how to prepare for your thyroid blood test, and much more. "Test Your Thyroid Function" is an indispensable resource for anyone looking to thoroughly understand and take control of their metabolic health.

Benedicte Mai Lerche MSc PhD

Causes of Slow Metabolism

Dr. Ray Peat identified several factors that can lead to slow metabolism. Three common causes include inadequate secretion of thyroid hormones by the thyroid gland (Sluggish Gland), ineffective conversion of T4 to active thyroid hormone T3 (Conversion Defect), or impaired cellular response to T3 (T3 Blockage) (Peat R., Generative Energy, 2001a, pp. 72-74; Wilson, 2015, pp. 24-28).

Dr. Ray Peat's extensive research suggests that hypothyroidism usually arises from a combination of these factors. Regardless of the underlying cause, hypothyroidism ultimately leads to a deficiency of biological energy (ATP) (Peat R., Generative Energy, 2001a, pp. 2-3; Peat R., TSH, temperature, pulse rate, and other indicators in hypothyroidism, 2008a).

A sluggish thyroid gland:

An underactive thyroid gland is unable to produce sufficient amounts of the thyroid hormones T4 and T3. This deficiency might be attributed to the gland's intrinsic limitations.

However, other factors such as a diet high in polyunsaturated fats, undercooked cruciferous vegetables like raw cabbage, and excess estrogen can also contribute to reducing the hormonal output of the thyroid gland (Peat R., From PMS to Menopause: Female Hormones in Context, 2001b, pp. 155-156).

Estrogen is primarily regarded as a female hormone, but men produce it as well. According to Dr. Ray Peat, controlled amounts of estrogen are essential for female ovulation and pregnancy (Peat R., From PMS to Menopause: Female Hormones in Context, 2001b, pp. 3-22).

However, excessive estrogen from endogenous sources (produced by the body) or exogenous sources (such as food or birth control pills) can have many negative effects. Dr. Peat explains that estrogen excess has a shock-like effect and contributes to stress, inflammation, aging, and hypothyroidism (Peat R., From PMS to Menopause: Female Hormones in Context, 2001b, pp. 3-22).

Food sources high in estrogen include beans, soybeans, lentils, and beer, among others (Medical News Today, 2023b; Peat R., Natural estrogens, 2008b)

Conversion defect:

Sometimes, people have high levels of T4 yet still experience symptoms of slow metabolism. This situation likely occurs due to inefficient conversion of the storage hormone T4 to the active thyroid T3 (Peat R., Generative Energy, 2001a, p. 74).

As previously noted, the liver is the primary organ responsible for converting T4 to T3. Consequently, compromised liver function can lead to hypothyroidism (Peat R., Generative Energy, 2001a, p. 73).

Typically, women have less robust liver function compared to men, in part due to the adverse effects of estrogen on liver activity. Consequently, this makes the conversion of T4 to T3 more challenging for women (Peat R., Generative Energy, 2001a, p. 74). Many foods also have estrogenic properties.

Factors such as a diet lacking in high-quality protein and B vitamins can also impair liver function, subsequently limiting the production of T3. (Ray Peat Clips, 2016e).

Low blood sugar (hypoglycemia) and a lack of selenium are also known to impede the liver's ability to convert T4 to T3 (Peat R., Generative Energy, 2001a, pp. 73-75; Wilson, 2015, p. 26).

The production of T3 is further compromised by physical or mental stress, as stress hormones (cortisol and adrenaline) directly interfere with the T4 to T3 conversion process (Peat R., TSH, temperature, pulse rate, and other indicators in hypothyroidism, 2008a, p. 3)

T3 blockage:

Dr. Ray Peat emphasized that even if an individual produces sufficient levels of T3, they may still experience symptoms of slow metabolism. This can be attributed to decreased tissue sensitivity to T3, for example, from a diet high in polyunsaturated fats (Peat R., Generative Energy, 2001a, p. 72).

Another reason can be the production of reverse T3, also known as rT3, which is an inactive form of T3 that acts as a metabolic suppressor by chemically inhibiting the activity of the active thyroid hormone T3 (Peat R., Nutrition for Women: 100 Short Articles, 2001d, p. 20; Peat R., TSH, temperature, pulse rate, and other indicators in hypothyroidism, 2008a).

Stress, and specifically the stress hormones adrenaline and cortisol, can increase the production of rT3, thereby undermining thyroid function at the cellular level (Peat R., TSH, temperature, pulse rate, and other indicators in hypothyroidism, 2008a, p. 3; Ray Peat Clips, 2016a).

The body is known to ramp up the production of rT3 during crises such as critical illness, extreme dieting, or starvation (Mary Shomon, 2022; Alan Jacobs, 2023).

This book thoroughly explores how diet impacts metabolism. The wrong diet can suppress metabolism through several of the factors described above.

Regardless of the specific underlying cause, a slow metabolic rate ultimately leads to a deficiency of biological energy (ATP), manifesting in symptoms of slow metabolism (hypothyroidism) (Peat R., Generative Energy, 2001a, pp. 72-74; Peat R., TSH, temperature, pulse rate, and other indicators in hypothyroidism, 2008a).

Table 1.1 lists factors that suppress the metabolic rate, providing a reference for later discussions.

Factors That Suppress Metabolism	
Estrogen from natural, synthetic, or environmental sources.	Excess estrogen inhibits the secretion of thyroid hormones from the gland, which can lead to goiter (enlargement of the thyroid gland). Excess estrogen also interferes with liver function, and its ability to convert T4 to T3.
A diet high in polyunsaturated fats (PUFAs)	PUFAs block the release of thyroid hormones from the thyroid gland, hinder the transport of these hormones in the blood, and inhibit the tissue's response to the active thyroid hormone T3.
Foods high in carotenes	Carotenes block thyroid function in the same way as PUFAs. Carrot juice, cooked carrots, and sweet potatoes contain large amounts of carotene.
B-Vitamin deficiency	A lack of B vitamins impairs liver function and thereby hinders the conversion of T4 to T3.
Lack of protein	A diet low in high-quality protein impairs liver function

	and thereby hinders the conversion of T4 to T3.
Lack of selenium, iodine, and copper	A deficiency in these trace minerals can impede metabolism in multiple ways. The optimal source for these minerals is a weekly serving of shellfish.
Too much iodine	Excessive iodine from supplements or iodinated salt can lead to inflammation of the thyroid gland.
High-stress hormones	Stress, whether mental or physical, directly inhibits the conversion of T4 to T3. Fasting and low blood sugar increase stress levels.
Reverse T3	Reverse T3 blocks the tissue's response to the active thyroid hormone T3. Stress and dieting can increase the production of Reverse T3.
Low blood sugar	Low blood sugar inhibits the liver enzyme activity that converts T4 into T3 low blood sugar also leads to an increase in stress hormones.

Raw vegetables from the cabbage Family	These cruciferous vegetables contain goitrogens, which impair the synthesis of thyroid hormones by the thyroid gland.
The amino acids cysteine, methionine, and tryptophan	These amino acids, found in large amounts in muscle meat, have anti-metabolic properties.
Amygdalin	Amygdalin, a compound found in many nuts, seeds, and grains, inhibits thyroid function.
High PTH	Parathyroid hormone (PTH) has antimetabolic effects. A diet high in phosphate and low in calcium will increase the secretion of PTH.

Table 1.1 List of factors that suppress metabolism: Diet can affect the metabolic rate directly by inhibiting thyroid function at different levels, or indirectly by causing physiological changes that negatively impact the metabolic rate.

What Triggers Slow Metabolism?

Based on my work with clients and personal experience with hypothyroidism, I've observed that a slow metabolic rate is often triggered by anti-metabolic dietary choices and different forms of stress, whether mental or physical.

According to Dr. Ray Peat, many health-conscious individuals may unintentionally make lifestyle choices that hinder their metabolism. These choices can include engaging in stressful, strenuous exercises and consuming foods such as soybeans, beans, lentils, nuts, polyunsaturated fats, and undercooked cruciferous vegetables like broccoli, cauliflower, and cabbage, all of which are known to negatively impact thyroid function (Peat R., Generative Energy, 2001a, p. 75).

While some individuals may have a history of mildly low metabolism, significant issues often do not manifest until they adopt an anti-metabolic diet or encounter specific stressors.

Dr. Ray Peat's nutritional research stands out from other diets as a comprehensive pro-metabolic system based on a deep understanding of the body's biochemical functions. With over 50 years dedicated to studying the interactions between nutrition and metabolism, Dr. Peat developed a diet specifically designed to support thyroid function and combat stress, inflammation, and premature aging.

These dietary principles are essential for those diagnosed with hypothyroidism and anyone seeking to optimize their metabolic rate.

This book thoroughly collects and explains Dr. Peat's dietary principles, enabling you to implement this unique pro-metabolic diet system into your daily life.

It will reveal how many foods commonly considered healthy by doctors and nutritionists can actually harm your metabolism. Additionally, you will discover that many foods labeled as unhealthy are, in fact, beneficial for supporting a healthy metabolism, reducing inflammation, and combating stress and aging.

The following chapter will delve into Dr. Ray Peat's research on fats, and what you learn may be shocking but true. Be ready to change your diet forever.

Chapter 2: Fats

Benedicte Mai Lerche MSc PhD

A New Perspective on Fats

One major change you'll encounter when adopting the "Ray Peat diet" involves the types of fats you consume.

Health guidelines commonly advocate for the intake of polyunsaturated fats found in various liquid cooking oils, including corn, canola, soy, safflower, sunflower, flaxseed, sesame, peanut, and almond oils (Peat R., Unsaturated Vegetable Oils: Toxic, 2006a).

Conversely, Dr. Ray Peat emphasized the importance of avoiding polyunsaturated fats. He advocated for the consumption of saturated fats such as coconut oil and butter instead (Peat R., From PMS to Menopause: Female Hormones in Context, 2001b, p. 157).

Dr. Peat pointed out that diets high in polyunsaturated fats are linked to numerous health issues, such as abnormal blood clotting, inflammation, immune deficiency, shock, accelerated aging, digestive disturbances, obesity, and a slow metabolic rate, which is the main topic of this book (Peat R., From PMS to Menopause: Female Hormones in Context, 2001b, pp. 153-161;

Peat R., Fats and degeneration, 2009a; Peat R., Unsaturated Vegetable Oils: Toxic, 2006a).

Additionally, Dr. Peat noted that polyunsaturated fats increase estrogen levels in the body and have direct estrogenic properties themselves (Peat R., Unsaturated fatty acids: Nutritionally essential, or toxic?, 2007b). Estrogen is as mentioned, a potent thyroid suppressor.

Dr. Ray Peat explained that saturated fats, such as butter and coconut oil, do not contribute to arteriosclerosis or heart disease (Peat R., Unsaturated Vegetable Oils: Toxic, 2006a). Instead, they offer protection against the harmful effects of polyunsaturated fats, thereby supporting metabolism and providing several health benefits, including anti-stress, anti-inflammatory, anti-fibrotic, and germicidal properties (Peat R., From PMS to Menopause: Female Hormones in Context, 2001b, pp. 153-161; Peat R., Cholesterol, longevity, intelligence, and health., 2007a; Peat R., Fats and degeneration, 2009a; Peat R., Coconut Oil, 2006b; Peat R., Fats, functions & malfunctions, 2013; Functional performance Systems, 2012b).

Polyunsaturated fats are not solely confined to liquid cooking oils; they are found in varying amounts across all types of food. Given their ubiquity, it is impossible to adopt a diet that is entirely free from these fatty acids.

The key is to minimize PUFA intake as much as possible and to incorporate saturated fats into your daily diet to counteract the adverse effects of the small amounts of PUFAs that will inevitably remain, even with diligent efforts to reduce them. Dr. Ray Peat emphasizes that the harm from PUFAs stems not from their quantity but from the ratio of these fats to saturated fats (Peat R., Unsaturated Vegetable Oils: Toxic, 2006a).

Understanding Dr. Peat's advice on fats can be challenging due to its direct contradiction with mainstream health recommendations.

This chapter explores the relationship between fats and health, emphasizing the risks associated with polyunsaturated fats and the significant benefits of switching to saturated fats for optimal metabolism and overall health.

To fully grasp why the types of fats in your diet are so significant, it's essential to understand their distinct chemical structures. The structural differences between saturated and polyunsaturated fats lead to their vastly different biological effects, which will be the focus of the next section.

The Structure of Fats

When discussing "fat," we commonly refer to sources such as butter, coconut oil, olive oil, and other vegetable oils like corn and soybean oil, as well as animal-derived fats including pork fat (lard) and beef fat (tallow) (Open Oregon, 2020g).

Additionally, it's important to note that nearly all foods contain some fats. Milk products, cheese, meat, oily fish, nuts, seeds, and grains all contain significant amounts of fat. Even vegetables contain a small quantity of fat (Henrik Parbo, 2015; Peat R., Unsaturated Vegetable Oils: Toxic, 2006a; Open Oregon, 2020g).

Structurally fats are built up of molecules called triglycerides, consisting of three fatty acids bonded to a glycerol backbone, see Figure 2.1 (Henrik Parbo, 2015; Study Mind, 2024; Open Oregon, 2020e).

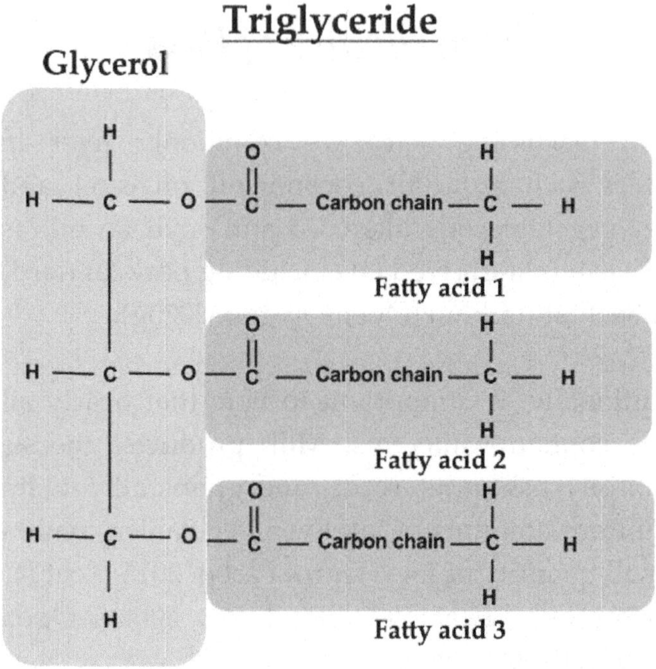

Triglyceride

Glycerol

Figure 2.1: The structure of a triglyceride, showing the glycerol backbone and three attached fatty acids (Open Oregon, 2020g).

A fatty acid is composed of long chains of carbon atoms with hydrogen atoms attached. There are various fatty acids found in nature; for some examples, see Figure 2.2 (Henrik Parbo, 2015).

Fatty acids vary based on the length of the carbon chain and the degree of saturation (Open Oregon, 2020g).

The term "saturation" refers to whether the carbon atoms are filled ("saturated") to capacity with hydrogen atoms. In a saturated fatty acid, the carbon chain is completely filled with hydrogens, resulting in only single bonds between the carbons. However, each time two hydrogens are missing, it leads to a double bond in the carbon chain (point of unsaturation) (Henrik Parbo, 2015; Open Oregon, 2020f).

Fatty acids are classified into three main categories based on the degree of saturation, refer to Figure 2.2 for illustrations (Khan Academy, 2024; Saini RK, 2021):

Saturated Fatty Acids: The carbon chain is fully saturated with hydrogen atoms, featuring only single bonds between the carbon atoms.

Monounsaturated Fatty Acids (MUFAs): Removing two hydrogen atoms results in a carbon chain with one double bond (one point of unsaturation).

Polyunsaturated Fatty Acids (PUFAs): The absence of more hydrogen atoms, leads to a carbon chain with two or more double bonds (two or more points of unsaturation).

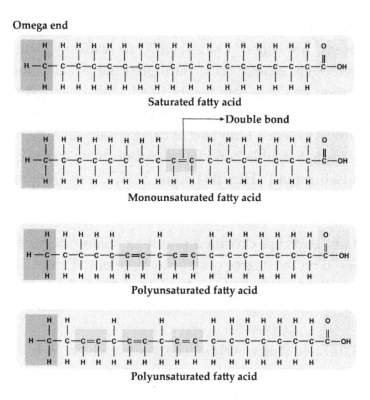

Figure 2.2: *The structures of a saturated, monounsaturated, and polyunsaturated fatty acid (Open Oregon, 2020f).*

The different types of fats originate from the variations in fatty acids present in their triglycerides (Study Mind, 2024; Open Oregon, 2020f; Henrik Parbo, 2015).

Some fats are primarily composed of saturated fatty acids, while others are rich in polyunsaturated fatty acids (PUFAs) or monounsaturated fatty acids (MUFAs) (Open Oregon, 2020f).

Figure 2.3 illustrates the distribution of saturated, monounsaturated, and polyunsaturated fatty acids in some common fats (Open Oregon, 2020f).

Coconut oil, butter, beef fat, and cacao butter (the fat found in chocolate) are categorized as saturated fats because they mainly contain saturated fatty acids. It is important to note that they still include small quantities of harmful PUFAs (Open Oregon, 2020f). This means that completely avoiding PUFAs is practically impossible.

On the other hand, many commonly recommended vegetable oils have a high proportion of polyunsaturated fatty acids (PUFAs), which is why they should be avoided if you wish to have a diet low in PUFAs (Henrik Parbo, 2015; Peat R., From PMS to Menopause: Female Hormones in Context, 2001b, pp. 153-161).

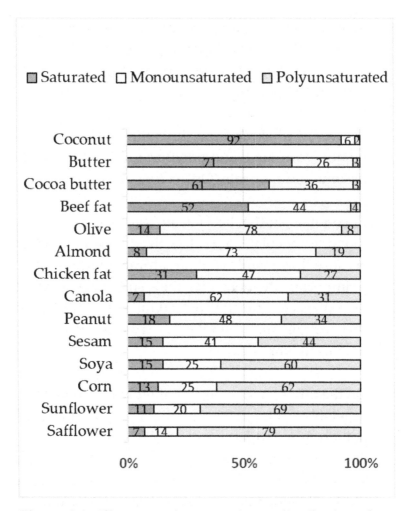

Figure **2.3:** *Illustrates the approximate distribution of saturated, monounsaturated, and polyunsaturated fatty acids found in common fats and oils (Centra food, 2024; Iowa State University Extension and Outreach, 2019).*

Aren't PUFAs Essential Fats?

Polyunsaturated fatty acids (PUFAs) from food can be divided into two main groups—omega-3 and omega-6—based on the location of the first double bond when counting from the end of the carbon chain, also referred to as the "omega" end (Saini RK, 2021; Harvard Medical School, 2022; Open Oregon, 2020f; Sokoła-Wysoczańska, 2018).

Omega end

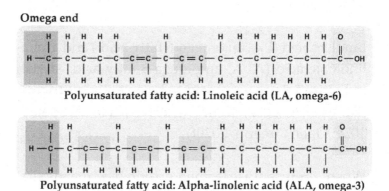

Polyunsaturated fatty acid: Linoleic acid (LA, omega-6)

Polyunsaturated fatty acid: Alpha-linolenic acid (ALA, omega-3)

Figure 2.4: The two "so-called" essential fatty acids, linoleic acid (LA, an omega-6) and alpha-linolenic acid (ALA, an omega-3) are shown here (Open Oregon, 2020f).

Fatty acids with the first double bond at the third carbon from the omega end are called omega-3 fatty acids. Those with the first double bond at the sixth carbon from the omega end are known as omega-6 fatty acids. See Figure 2.4 for examples (Linus Pauling Institute, 2024; Open Oregon, 2020f).

Both omega-3 and omega-6 fatty acids are commonly endorsed as healthy fats by health professionals and the media (Open Oregon, 2020f). This viewpoint sharply contrasts with Dr. Ray Peat's recommendation to avoid all polyunsaturated fatty acids (PUFAs), including both omega-3 and omega-6 fatty acids.

Linoleic acid (LA, an omega-6 fatty acid) and alpha-linolenic acid (ALA, an omega-3 fatty acid) shown in Figure 2.4 are even said to be essential nutrients, (Farag MA, 2022; Kaur N, 2014; Khan Academy, 2024; Open Oregon, 2020f)

When a nutrient is deemed essential, it means that the body requires it for good health, but cannot produce it on its own, so it must be obtained through the diet (Linus Pauling Institute, 2024).

The belief that polyunsaturated fatty acids (PUFAs) are healthy fats is closely linked to the widespread notion of essential fatty acids.

The concept of essential fatty acids originates from research conducted in the early 1900s by a husband-and-wife team George and Mildred Burr (American Society for Biochemistry and Molecular Biology, 2012).

In 1929 the Burrs published a paper explaining that linoleic acid (LA) cured several symptoms including a skin condition with dermatitis and dandruff, in their experimental rats (Peat R., Unsaturated fatty acids: Nutritionally essential, or toxic?, 2007b).

The Burrs claimed that linoleic acid (LA) was an essential nutrient and coined the phrase "essential fatty acids" (American Society for Biochemistry and Molecular Biology, 2012)".

Dr. Ray Peat explained, that in 1929, most of the B vitamins and essential trace minerals were unknown to nutritionists. He pointed out that various nutritional deficiencies, including deficiency of vitamin B6, trace minerals, and biotin produce symptoms similar to those observed by the Burrs (Peat R., Fats and degeneration, 2009a; Peat R., Unsaturated fatty acids: Nutritionally essential, or toxic?, 2007b).

He further clarified that the observations made by the Burrs can be explained by the fact that PUFAs significantly suppress the metabolic rate, thereby reducing the need for vitamins and minerals. Essentially, the Burrs resolved a nutrient deficiency by inhibiting the metabolic rate with PUFAs (Ray Peat Clips, 2016b; Peat R., Unsaturated fatty acids: Nutritionally essential, or toxic?, 2007b).

Despite the existence of studies that disprove the conclusion of the Burrs, their 1929 paper is often cited as proof that PUFAs are essential nutrients (Peat R., Unsaturated fatty acids: Nutritionally essential, or toxic?, 2007b; Peat R., Fats and degeneration, 2009a).

In contrast, Dr. Ray Peat strongly emphasized that none of the PUFAs including linoleic acid (LA), and alpha-linolenic acid (ALA), are essential nutrients (Peat R., Unsaturated Vegetable Oils: Toxic, 2006a).

Foods high in PUFAs (omega-3 and omega-6 fatty acids) are frequently advertised as healthy and claimed to offer protection against arteriosclerosis, heart disease, and inflammation, among other benefits (Health Line, 2023).

Contrary to these claims, Dr. Ray Peat argued that PUFAs (omega-3 and omega-6 fatty acids) do not offer health benefits. He explained that the numerous double bonds in these fatty acids render them extremely harmful to your metabolism and general health (Peat R., Unsaturated Vegetable Oils: Toxic, 2006a; Peat R., Fats, functions & malfunctions, 2013).

There are three main types of damage from PUFAs: First, they inhibit thyroid function, meaning a diet high in PUFAs significantly slows the metabolic rate. Second, PUFAs impair the immune system. Third, PUFAs readily form free radicals, which damage cells in various ways (Peat R., From PMS to Menopause: Female Hormones in Context, 2001b, pp. 156-157).

Consequently, a diet rich in PUFAs contributes to many of the problems they are purported to alleviate (Peat R., Unsaturated fatty acids: Nutritionally essential, or toxic?, 2007b; Peat R., Fats and degeneration, 2009a)

In the next section, I will detail the serious health dangers of a diet high in PUFAs.

Benedicte Mai Lerche MSc PhD

Health Dangers of PUFAs

The structural distinctions between saturated and polyunsaturated fats account for their markedly different biological impacts. According to Dr. Peat, an excess of PUFAs harms all body systems (Peat R., From PMS to Menopause: Female Hormones in Context, 2001b, pp. 153-161).

PUFAs inhibit proteolytic enzymes:

PUFAs inhibit enzymes that break down proteins (proteolytic enzymes). These enzymes are essential not only for digestion but also for the production of thyroid hormones, clot removal, immunity, and overall cellular adaptability. The inhibition of proteolytic enzymes increases the risks of abnormal blood clotting, inflammation, immune deficiency, shock, aging, and obesity. Because PUFAs impair protein digestion in the stomach, it is possible to become malnourished on a high PUFA diet (Peat R., Unsaturated Vegetable Oils: Toxic, 2006a).

PUFAs go rancid and damage cells:

The numerous double bonds in PUFAs create an open structure that renders these molecules unstable. When ingested, PUFAs are exposed to the body's warm, oxygen-rich environment, leading to their rancidity. This process of spontaneous oxidation generates free radicals (Peat R., Unsaturated Vegetable Oils: Toxic, 2006a).

Free radicals are reactive molecular fragments that damage cells and contribute to cellular aging (Peat R., Unsaturated Vegetable Oils: Toxic, 2006a; Dynamic Science, 2024).

The free radicals can impair enzymes and other cellular components, particularly affecting the cells' ability to produce biological energy (ATP). They may also interact with cellular structures like DNA and proteins, potentially binding to them and causing structural and functional abnormalities (Peat R., Unsaturated Vegetable Oils: Toxic, 2006a).

Since the spontaneous oxidation of polyunsaturated fatty acids (PUFAs) is accelerated by heat, it is commonly recommended not to use PUFA-rich oils for high-heat cooking. Instead, more stable fats like coconut oil and butter are recommended, as saturated fats, which lack double bonds, are more resistant to oxidation when heated (Doctor, Diet, 2024a).

Expanding on this guidance, Dr. Ray Peat advises against the consumption of highly polyunsaturated oils entirely. He highlights that PUFAs are extremely unstable, even without heating, and their detrimental effects on health make their consumption in any form ill-advised (Peat R., Unsaturated Vegetable Oils: Toxic, 2006a).

PUFAs suppress the immune system:

Fish oils, which are rich in omega-3 fatty acids are often promoted for their anti-inflammatory effects. However, Dr. Ray Peat argued that this is due to the immunosuppressive properties of fish oils, which might appear beneficial initially but can have detrimental effects over time (Peat R., The Great Fish Oil Experiment, 2007c). Similarly, vegetable oils rich in polyunsaturated fatty acids (PUFAs) are known for their immune-suppressing effects. When emulsified with water for intravenous injection, these PUFA-rich oils are specifically marketed to suppress the immune system in organ transplant patients. Additionally, PUFAs have been shown to directly destroy white blood cells (Peat R., Unsaturated Vegetable Oils: Toxic, 2006a).

PUFA suppresses thyroid function:

Dr. Ray Peat strongly emphasized that PUFAs inhibit thyroid function, leading to significant metabolic suppression. This effect occurs at various levels (Peat R., From PMS to Menopause: Female Hormones in Context, 2001b, p. 178; Peat R., Unsaturated Vegetable Oils: Toxic, 2006a; Peat R., Nutrition for Women: 100 Short Articles, 2001d, p. iii):

PUFAs block the secretion of thyroid hormones (T4 and T3) from the thyroid gland (Peat R., From PMS to Menopause: Female Hormones in Context, 2001b, p. 155; Peat R., Unsaturated Vegetable Oils: Toxic, 2006a).

PUFAs also interfere with the transport of thyroid hormones in the bloodstream by hindering their binding to carrier proteins (Peat R., Fats, functions & malfunctions, 2013; Peat R., From PMS to Menopause: Female Hormones in Context, 2001b, pp. 177-178).

Additionally, PUFAs inhibit the cellular response to the active thyroid hormone, T3 (Peat R., Nutrition for Women: 100 Short Articles, 2001d, p. iii; Peat R., From PMS to Menopause: Female Hormones in Context, 2001b, pp. 177-178).

This means that PUFA acts as a powerful suppressor of thyroid function at all levels leading to a state of slow metabolic rate (Peat R., Unsaturated Vegetable Oils: Toxic, 2006a).

Additional research by scholars such as Altınterim (2012), Mamounis (2017), and Speakman (2024) has also shown that polyunsaturated fatty acids (PUFAs) suppress thyroid function and reduce the metabolic rate (Altınterim, 2012; Mamounis, 2017; Speakman, 2024).

Benedicte Mai Lerche MSc PhD

How Did PUFAs Become Food?

Fifty years ago, paints were primarily made from soy oil, safflower oil, and linseed (flaxseed) oil. However, when chemists developed methods to produce cheaper petroleum-based paints, the vast seed oil industry faced significant challenges in selling its products (Peat R., Unsaturated Vegetable Oils: Toxic, 2006a).

Simultaneously, farmers were seeking to enhance the fattening of their pigs while reducing feed costs. Corn and soybeans emerged as effective solutions. Consequently, the crops once grown for the paint industry found a new purpose as animal feed (Peat R., Unsaturated Vegetable Oils: Toxic, 2006a).

Subsequently, these same oils, effective in cheaply fattening animals, were marketed as human foods. However, attention from their fattening properties was directed to heart disease and "cholesterol." Tragically, this focus has persisted the longest, even after the unsaturated oils were proven to cause heart disease (Peat R., Unsaturated Vegetable Oils: Toxic, 2006a).

In the following, I will address the misconceptions surrounding saturated and polyunsaturated fats and their impact on cholesterol and heart disease.

The Cholesterol Myth

The vegetable oil industry has created a phobia about the consumption of saturated fats and cholesterol, but according to Dr. Ray Peat there is no basis for the idea that these foods should be avoided (Peat R., Generative Energy, 2001a, p. 17).

For over fifty years, the prevailing dietary advice has been to increase PUFAs and decrease saturated fats to lower cholesterol levels. It is recommended to avoid foods such as butter, cream, eggs, and red meat, which contain both saturated fat and cholesterol (Peat R., Cholesterol, longevity, intelligence, and health., 2007a).

The notion that cholesterol causes atherosclerosis and heart disease resurfaced in the 1950s when the vegetable oil industry realized that their polyunsaturated oils could lower serum cholesterol levels (Peat R., Cholesterol, longevity, intelligence, and health., 2007a).

Since then, the vegetable oil industry has been remarkably successful in convincing both the general population and medical professionals that cholesterol and saturated fats (which raise cholesterol) are harmful, while their polyunsaturated vegetable oils are healthy and heart-protective (Peat R., Cholesterol, longevity, intelligence, and health., 2007a; Peat R., Fats and degeneration, 2009a).

While it's true that highly polyunsaturated oils can lower serum cholesterol levels, they do so by exerting toxicity within the body. Dr. Peat highlighted that many other toxins also lower cholesterol, a fact that is often overlooked (Peat R., Cholesterol, longevity, intelligence, and health., 2007a).

In addition, it is crucial to recognize that cholesterol is not a harmful substance, but a life-essential molecule, serving as one of the most protective molecules in the human body (Peat R., Cholesterol, longevity, intelligence, and health., 2007a; Ravnskov, 2020).

Among its many protective effects, cholesterol serves as the building block for the body's anti-aging and anti-stress hormones: pregnenolone, progesterone, and dehydroepiandrosterone (DHEA) (Peat R., Generative Energy, 2001a, pp. 68-69).

It is essential to recognize that Dr. Peat, along with many other researchers, including the renowned cholesterol expert Dr. Uffe Ravnskov, strongly emphasized that cholesterol is a life-essential molecule that is not the cause of arteriosclerosis or heart disease (Rosch, 2008; Ravnskov, 2020; Ravnskov U d., 2018 ; Ravnskov U D., 2016). Instead, various inflammatory processes play a role in these conditions (Peat R., Cholesterol, longevity, intelligence, and health., 2007a; Rosch, 2008).

Benedicte Mai Lerche MSc PhD

Metabolism & Cholesterol

Dr. Ray Peat explained that high cholesterol levels naturally result from a slow metabolism. He emphasized that the only safe way to reduce cholesterol levels is by increasing the metabolic rate.

Elevated serum cholesterol is a well-documented symptom of hypothyroidism (Barnes & Galton, 1976). This inverse correlation between thyroid function and cholesterol levels occurs because the active thyroid hormone, T3, is essential for cholesterol utilization, which involves its conversion into the protective hormones pregnenolone, progesterone, and DHEA. When the metabolic rate is slow, cholesterol tends to accumulate because it is not being used to produce these protective hormones (Peat R., Generative Energy, 2001a, pp. 68-69).

Paradoxically, highly polyunsaturated vegetable oils, which are touted as beneficial for preventing atherosclerosis and heart disease, strongly inhibit thyroid function. This inhibition leads to increased cholesterol and reduced levels of pregnenolone, progesterone, and DHEA, making the body more vulnerable to stress, inflammation, and aging (Peat R., Unsaturated Vegetable Oils: Toxic, 2006a).

PUFAs Cause Obesity

Dr. Ray Peat emphasized a significant link between obesity and the consumption of polyunsaturated fatty acids (PUFAs) (Peat R., From PMS to Menopause: Female Hormones in Context, 2001b, pp. 177-178). This viewpoint is also supported by other researchers (Altınterim, 2012; Speakman, 2024).

According to Dr. Ray Peat, the typical American diet, which is high in PUFAs, leads to a metabolic rate approximately 25% lower than that of populations consuming diets predominantly based on saturated fats (Peat R., From PMS to Menopause: Female Hormones in Context, 2001b, p. 177).

It's important to recognize that the fatty acid composition of the body's fat stores, or adipose tissues, reflects the habitual diet. Therefore, if your diet is high in PUFAs, these fatty acids will be predominant in your fat tissues (The American Journal of Clinical Nutrition, 1980).

During periods of hunger or stress, the body releases fatty acids from its fat stores into the bloodstream to generate energy (Ray Peat Clips, 2016f). If the released fatty acids are polyunsaturated, they will suppress thyroid function and slow down the metabolic rate (Ray Peat Clips, 2017b; Peat R., Fats, functions & malfunctions, 2013; Ray Peat KMUD, 2008)

This creates a harmful cycle where a diet rich in PUFAs impairs thyroid function, which in turn slows the metabolic rate, resulting in increased fat storage and weight gain. As PUFAs accumulate in the fat tissues, they further inhibit thyroid function, leading to additional weight gain and more stored PUFAs. Essentially, the more polyunsaturated fats consumed, the more challenging it becomes to lose weight. This detrimental cycle is illustrated in Figure 2.5.

To break this vicious cycle, it's essential to shift towards a diet rich in saturated fats and avoid high-PUFA foods. This dietary change will gradually replace the stored PUFAs with saturated fatty acids, a process that can take up to four years depending on the amount of stored fat (Functional Performance Systems, 2012a).

Because the body prefers to burn saturated fats over PUFAs, there is a tendency to accumulate more PUFAs in fat tissue over time. This accumulation contributes to the natural decrease in metabolic rate that occurs with age. Therefore, it's crucial to consistently avoid PUFAs in your diet to maintain a healthier metabolic rate (Ray Peat Clips, 2017b; Ray Peat Clips, 2016f).

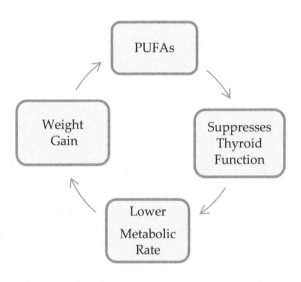

Figure 2.5: Illustration of the vicious cycle where polyunsaturated fatty acids (PUFAs) suppress thyroid function, leading to a lower metabolic rate. This results in increased weight gain and the accumulation of PUFAs in the body's fat tissues, which further suppresses thyroid function, perpetuating the cycle.

Benedicte Mai Lerche MSc PhD

Anti-Obesity Effects of Coconut Oil

Dr. Ray Peat explained that saturated fats help prevent obesity and specifically highlighted coconut oil for its ability to accelerate metabolism and aid in weight loss. This is due to coconut oil's high content of medium-chain fatty acids (MCT), which serve as an energy source that effectively protects tissues from the harmful effects of PUFAs and reduces their anti-thyroid impact (Peat R., Coconut Oil, 2006b; Peat R., Nutrition for Women: 100 Short Articles, 2001d, pp. II-IV).

When Dr. Peat began integrating coconut oil into his diet, he had already abstained from consuming PUFAs for quite some time. Initially, he started by consuming a daily tablespoon of coconut oil with his dinner. He noticed an immediate pro-metabolic effect lasting approximately two hours, characterized by a feeling of warmth, deeper breathing, a rosier complexion, and an elevated pulse rate of around 98 beats per minute. He observed this same response every day for a couple of weeks while digesting a small amount of coconut oil (Peat R., Coconut Oil, 2006b).

With continued use, the immediate pro-metabolic effect of the coconut oil waned, so Dr. Peat increased his daily consumption to about an ounce (two tablespoons). Over the subsequent six months, he observed a gradual decrease in his weight, amounting to a loss of approximately 15 pounds (7 kg), despite maintaining the same diet and adding 200 to 250 calories per day in the form of coconut oil (Peat R., Coconut Oil, 2006b; Peat R., Nutrition for Women: 100 Short Articles, 2001d, pp. II-IV).

According to Dr. Peat, the anti-obesity effect of coconut oil is evident in both animal experiments and in individuals who regularly incorporate it into their diet (Peat R., Coconut Oil, 2006b).

Dr. Peat emphasized that the health benefits of coconut oil extend beyond its anti-obesity effect, offering protection against stress, heart disease, excessive blood clotting, sun damage, and premature aging, among other conditions (Peat R., Nutrition for Women: 100 Short Articles, 2001d, pp. II-IV). Due to its numerous health advantages, coconut oil should be considered an integral part of a protective pro-metabolic diet (Peat R., Coconut Oil, 2006b; Peat R., Unsaturated Vegetable Oils: Toxic, 2006a).

Different types of coconut oil:

There are two types of coconut oil: unrefined and refined coconut oil (Healthline, 2023). Unrefined coconut oil, sometimes called virgin coconut oil, is pressed from coconut meat and undergoes no further processing. It possesses a distinct coconut flavor (Healthline, 2023). Dr. Ray Peat often mentions its suitability for desserts, baking, homemade ice cream, and other dishes where the coconut taste is a pleasant addition.

However, it is important to understand that the aromatic compounds in unrefined coconut oil can cause allergic reactions in some individuals (Jodellefit, 2020). Therefore Dr. Peat recommended using refined coconut oil, which is taste-neutral. This oil undergoes additional processing steps to create a flavorless and odorless product (Healthline, 2023; Jodellefit, 2020).

It is important to mention that various fractions of coconut oil are increasingly being utilized as treatments for diseases, essentially being marketed as "drugs" (Peat R., From PMS to Menopause: Female Hormones in Context, 2001b, pp. 177-179).

In the fractionation process, different fatty acids are separated from the coconut oil (Glanbia

Nutritionals, 2024). Butyric acid is promoted for cancer treatment, lauric and myristic acids for viral infections, and medium-chain fatty acids (MCT) for weight loss (Peat R., From PMS to Menopause: Female Hormones in Context, 2001b, pp. 177-179).

It is important to note that pure MCT oil is acceptable within the "Ray Peat diet" framework and is also a widely used solvent in numerous nutritional supplements. Although many individuals tolerate MCT oil well, some may suffer from severe digestive and allergic reactions to this oil. For those affected, it is essential to avoid MCT oil (Ray Peat Clips, 2016d).

Dr. Peat emphasizes that while purification may enhance certain effects, fractionated products of coconut oil have not been used long enough to confidently assess their safety, which suggests that consuming whole refined coconut oil as a regular part of one's diet is the safest approach (Peat R., Coconut Oil, 2006b).

Test for Good and Bad Fats

The texture of fats is closely related to their degree of saturation (Henrik Parbo, 2015).

A simple refrigerator test can help you distinguish between highly saturated fats and those with a high content of PUFAs (Open Oregon, 2020f).

The melting temperature of fat decreases as the number of double bonds in its fatty acids increases. Therefore, highly polyunsaturated fats (oils) remain liquid at refrigerator temperatures, while highly saturated fats stay solid under the same conditions (Henrik Parbo, 2015).

Fat sources with a high percentage of saturated fatty acids, such as coconut oil and butter, are completely solid at refrigerator temperatures. This solidity is due to the lack of double bonds in saturated fatty acids, which makes them very straight, allowing them to pack tightly together, forming a compact structure that increases the melting temperature (Open Oregon, 2020f).

Conversely, fat sources rich in polyunsaturated fatty acids (PUFAs), such as corn, soy, and cottonseed oils, remain liquid at refrigerator temperatures. The many double bonds in polyunsaturated fatty acids introduce bends in the carbon chains, preventing the fatty acids from packing tightly together. This creates an open structure that lowers the melting temperature (Open Oregon, 2020f).

Interestingly, olive oil lies somewhere between saturated and polyunsaturated fats. It becomes thicker and clumpier in the refrigerator, indicating its unique composition. With about 10% polyunsaturated fatty acids, moderate consumption of olive oil is considered safe. Ray Peat recommends limiting intake to no more than 1-2 teaspoons daily (Peat R. , Unsaturated Vegetable Oils: Toxic, 2006a)

In summary, it is crucial to avoid all fats (oils) that remain liquid in the refrigerator, as these are highly polyunsaturated. Dr. Ray Peat recommends consuming healthy saturated fats such as coconut oil, butter, ghee, tallow (beef fat), and cocoa butter, which all remain solid at refrigerator temperatures.

From PUFAs to Saturated Fats

In this chapter, I've detailed the importance of avoiding PUFAs (omega-3 and omega-6 fatty acids). You have learned that vegetable oils like corn, canola, soy, safflower, sunflower, flaxseed, sesame, peanut, and almond oil are rich in PUFAs and that these oils are notably liquid at refrigeration temperatures due to their high unsaturation levels (Peat R., Unsaturated Vegetable Oils: Toxic, 2006a; Open Oregon, 2020f). However, it's crucial to acknowledge that PUFAs are also present in many other foods.

Fish oils are, as mentioned, abundant in omega-3 fatty acids. This means that oily fish such as salmon, mackerel, sardines, herring, anchovies, and tuna, as well as all forms of fish oil supplements, should be avoided (Peat R., The Great Fish Oil Experiment, 2007c).

The common classification of lard (pig fat) as "saturated fat" is misleading when pigs are fed a diet high in PUFAs from corn and soy. Non-ruminant animals such as pigs and poultry accumulate polyunsaturated fats from their diets in their tissues. Therefore, it is essential to avoid or at least restrict the consumption of fats and meats from nonruminants unless it is confirmed that they haven't been fed a diet rich in PUFAs. In contrast, the fats and meats from ruminant animals like beef and lamb are very saturated, making these a preferable dietary choice (Ray Peat Clips, 2016g).

Additionally, seeds, grains, almonds, avocados, and most nuts are also rich sources of PUFAs (Open Oregon, 2020f)

It's also important to recognize that even vegetables contain small amounts of PUFAs and that highly saturated fats like coconut oil and butter comprise about 1-3% PUFAs (Saventes, 2022).

This underscores that completely avoiding PUFAs is impossible unless the food is specially prepared in a laboratory setting (Peat R., Unsaturated Vegetable Oils: Toxic, 2006a).

The key strategy is to minimize PUFA intake as much as possible and include saturated fats in your daily diet to counteract the adverse effects of the small amounts of PUFAs. Dr. Ray Peat emphasizes that the harm from PUFAs is not due to their overall quantity but rather the ratio of these fats to saturated fats (Peat R., Unsaturated Vegetable Oils: Toxic, 2006a).

Dr. Peat highlighted coconut oil's unique properties for promoting weight loss. Other healthy saturated fats include butter, ghee, and cocoa butter—the fat found in chocolate. Saturated fats are also prevalent in dairy products and in the fat from ruminant animals (tallow). Safe saturated fats are identifiable by their solid state at refrigerator temperatures (Peat R., Unsaturated Vegetable Oils: Toxic, 2006a; Henrik Parbo, 2015; Peat R., Unsaturated fatty acids: Nutritionally essential, or toxic?, 2007b).

Due to their lack of double bonds, saturated fats do not suppress thyroid function or immune function, and because they are highly stable molecules, they do not easily go rancid as PUFAs do (Peat R., Unsaturated Vegetable Oils: Toxic, 2006a; Peat R., Unsaturated fatty acids: Nutritionally essential, or toxic?, 2007b).

Moreover, no fixed amount of saturated fats is recommended for daily consumption.

Key Points – Fats:

Saturated fats predominantly contain fatty acids without double bonds.

Polyunsaturated fats (PUFAs) predominantly contain fatty acids with two or more double bonds.

Saturated fats are solid at refrigerator temperature. PUFAs are liquid at refrigerator temperature and are therefore called oils.

PUFAs are grouped into omega-3 and omega-6 fatty acids – none of these are essential.

PUFAs go rancid, harm the immune system, suppress thyroid function, and cause obesity.

Saturated fats do not go rancid and are stable even at higher cooking temperatures. Saturated fats protect against the harm from PUFAs.

PUFAs lower cholesterol, but cholesterol is not the cause of heart disease.

Saturated fats do not cause arteriosclerosis or heart disease.

List of Bad & Good Fats

Bad Fats:

(Oils &Foods high in PUFAs)

- Oils that stay liquid in the refrigerator
- Seeds, nuts, grains, almonds, and peanuts
- Oily fish and fish oil supplements
- Fats from non-ruminant animals (pigs, poultry, etc.)

Good Fats:

(Fats and foods high in saturated fatty acids)

- Fats that stay solid in the refrigerator
- Refined coconut oil (taste neutral)
- Butter, clarified butter, ghee
- Extra-virgin olive oil (max 1-2 teaspoons daily)
- Cocoa butter
- Fats from ruminant animals (tallow)
- Fats from milk products and cheese

Benedicte Mai Lerche MSc PhD

Chapter 3: Carbohydrates

Benedicte Mai Lerche MSc PhD

A Different View on Carbohydrates

Carbohydrates are present in a wide variety of foods, including honey, table sugar, vegetables, rice, pasta, bread, breakfast cereals, and dairy products, which contain milk sugar (Open Oregon, 2020b).

Once ingested, these carbohydrates are broken down and converted into glucose. The concentration of glucose in the bloodstream is commonly referred to as blood sugar (Medline Plus, 2024; Open Oregon, 2020c).

Some carbohydrates convert to glucose quickly, causing rapid spikes and subsequent drops in blood sugar levels. Others break down more slowly, resulting in a gradual increase in glucose that helps maintain stable blood sugar levels over time (Open Oregon, 2020c; Peat R., Glycemia, starch, and sugar in context, 2009c).

Dr. Ray Peat has emphasized the importance of stable blood sugar levels in supporting a high metabolic rate. He noted that the liver requires a steady supply of glucose to convert the inactive thyroid hormone T4 into its active form, T3 (Peat R., Generative Energy, 2001a, pp. 73-74).

This chapter explores blood sugar regulation and the impact of different carbohydrates on blood sugar levels. With this understanding, you can select carbohydrates that best support your metabolism.

Additionally, the chapter challenges several common dietary beliefs. It explains why fasting can harm your metabolic rate and how low-carbohydrate diets, such as the ketogenic diet, may decrease T3 production.

You will learn about Dr. Ray Peat's preference for simple sugars, such as white sugar, honey, and sweet fruits, over starches like bread, pasta, and rice. The discussion also extends to the benefits of choosing refined products over whole grains. Furthermore, you will discover why raw vegetables, salads, and many high-fiber foods, often praised for their health benefits, might actually impair gut health and contribute to systemic inflammation.

To fully understand the various aspects of carbohydrates and their impact on your metabolic and overall health, it is crucial to comprehend their chemical structures, which will be the focus of the next section.

The Structure of Carbohydrates

Carbohydrates are composed of sugar molecules and are categorized into three primary groups: monosaccharides (single sugar molecules), disaccharides (two sugar molecules linked together), and polysaccharides (many sugar molecules linked together) (Open Oregon, 2020d)

Monosaccharides:

Monosaccharides are the simplest form of carbohydrates, consisting of single sugar molecules. Common examples include glucose, fructose, and galactose.

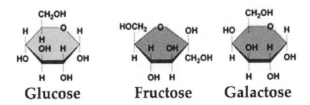

Glucose   Fructose   Galactose

Fig.3.1: *The chemical structures of the three monosaccharides — glucose, fructose, and galactose — are depicted.*

Disaccharides:

Sucrose, a sweet-tasting disaccharide found in fruits, honey, and table sugar, is composed of two monosaccharides, glucose and fructose, linked together (Open Oregon, 2020d).

Lactose, also known as milk sugar, is a sweet-tasting disaccharide found in dairy products. It consists of two monosaccharides, glucose and galactose, linked together. Dairy products are the only animal sources that contain significant amounts of carbohydrates, with the majority of our carbohydrates coming from plant-based foods (Open Oregon, 2020d)

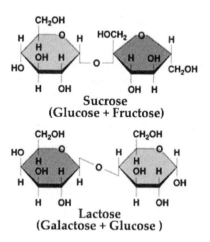

Figure 3.2: The chemical structures of the two disaccharides sucrose and lactose.

Polysaccharides:

Three types of polysaccharides, illustrated in Figure 3.3, are cellulose, starch, and glycogen. Each of these is made up of numerous glucose molecules linked together (Open Oregon, 2020d).

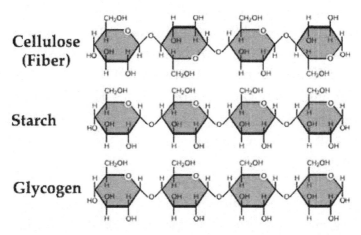

Figure 3.3: Shows the three polysaccharides cellulose, starch, and glycogen.

Cellulose, also known as dietary fiber, is found in whole plant foods such as whole grains, seeds, nuts, and fiber-rich fruits and vegetables. The bonds between the glucose molecules in cellulose cannot be broken down by human digestive enzymes, so we do not derive nutritional value from consuming fiber (Linus Pauling Institute, 2024; Open Oregon, 2020d). However, the gut bacteria in our large intestine can ferment some of these fibers, using them as food, which many researchers consider beneficial. This is why high-fiber foods are promoted for gut health (Open Oregon, 2020d; Open Oregon, 2020c)

Dr. Ray Peat recommended a few fiber-rich foods, but he also highlighted that many foods high in dietary fiber can pose issues by feeding and amplifying the presence of harmful bacteria within the gut. (Ray Peat Clips, 2016l) The dynamics between dietary fiber, gut bacteria, and intestinal health will be explored more deeply later in this chapter.

Starch which is found in foods such as bread, pasta, rice, and vegetables like potatoes is easily broken down by human digestive enzymes, whereby glucose is released into the bloodstream (Open Oregon, 2020d).

Glycogen, a polysaccharide synthesized by the human body, serves as our storage form of glucose. It is located in the liver and muscles and is drawn upon whenever blood sugar drops (Open Oregon, 2020d).

In this way, glycogen plays a crucial role in sustaining blood sugar levels during the night, between meals, or when fasting (Open Oregon, 2020d; National Council on Strength and Fitness, 2024).

Liver glycogen is converted into glucose, which then enters the bloodstream to supply energy to cells throughout the body. Meanwhile, glycogen stored in muscles fuels muscle activity exclusively. Both liver and muscle glycogen act as short-term energy reserves, collectively sustaining blood glucose levels for approximately 24 hours (Open Oregon, 2020d).

How carbohydrates affect the blood sugar:

When we consume carbohydrates in forms such as bread, pasta, rice, dairy, fruits, sugar, and honey, digestive enzymes break them down into monosaccharides, which eventually convert to glucose (Open Oregon, 2020c). The rate at which carbohydrates are converted into glucose affects their impact on blood sugar levels (Open Oregon, 2020c).

Starches are quickly digested, releasing glucose into the bloodstream and causing a significant spike in blood sugar levels (Open Oregon, 2020c).

In contrast, the galactose from lactose and the fructose from sucrose are converted into glucose more slowly. As a result, dairy, fruit, table sugar, and honey do not cause a sharp spike in blood sugar (Open Oregon, 2020c). Instead, these disaccharides help stabilize blood sugar levels, which is important for the production of T3 and, consequently, the metabolic rate.

Throughout this chapter, I will thoroughly explore the relationship between carbohydrates, blood sugar, and metabolism.

Importance of Stable Blood Sugar

Blood sugar is defined as the concentration of glucose in the bloodstream (Medline Plus, 2024; Open Oregon, 2020c).

Glucose is an essential nutrient that fuels the body, particularly crucial for the brain and nervous system, which are less efficient at using alternative energy sources. Glucose is also vital for metabolic health (Open Oregon, 2020d; Peat R., Generative Energy, 2001a, pp. 73-74).

The thyroid gland releases about three parts of thyroxine (T4) to one part of triiodothyronine (T3), allowing the liver to regulate thyroid function by converting more T4 to T3 when needed (Peat R., Generative Energy, 2001a, p. 73).

The amount of glucose in liver cells regulates the enzyme that converts T4 to T3 (Thyroid Patient Advocacy, 2024).

Conditions such as hypoglycemia (low blood sugar) or diabetes (where glucose isn't efficiently absorbed by cells) can lead to hypothyroidism due to the lack of glucose in the liver cells, which impairs the conversion of T4 to T3 (Thyroid Patient Advocacy, 2024).

Some people notice that their hands, feet, and nose get cold when they are hungry, and then warm up after eating. This is because the liver resumes forming T3 as blood sugar levels rise after a meal (Peat R., Generative Energy, 2001a, p. 74).

If someone has high T4 levels but shows symptoms of hypothyroidism, it may be because T4 isn't being converted to T3 by the liver. Dr. Ray Peat noted that dietary adjustments could help address this issue. Adding a piece of fruit or a glass of orange juice or milk between meals can stimulate the liver to produce more T3 (Peat R., Generative Energy, 2001a, pp. 73-74).

Dr. Peat advised against extended periods without food, recommending the consumption of small meals throughout the day to sustain T3 production. He even proposed a small meal of healthy carbohydrates before bedtime and highlighted the importance of beginning the day with beneficial carbohydrate sources, such as orange juice, to elevate blood glucose levels after the overnight fast (Thyroid Patient Advocacy, 2024; Peat R., Generative Energy, 2001a, pp. 73-74).

Experimental research indicates that incorporating an additional 200 to 300 calories of healthy carbohydrates into one's diet generally doesn't result in fat storage owing to the metabolic boost provided by healthy carbohydrates (Peat R., Generative Energy, 2001a, pp. 73-74). Throughout this chapter, you will learn what constitutes healthy carbohydrates according to Dr. Ray Peat.

Due to the importance of glucose, the body possesses inherent mechanisms aimed at maintaining stable blood sugar levels. In the next section, I will examine how the body responds to low blood sugar and how the metabolic rate is affected by these responses.

Benedicte Mai Lerche MSc PhD

The Stress of Low Blood Sugar

The body tries to keep the blood sugar/blood glucose level in a very narrow range between 60 to 150 mg/dl (Khan Academy, 2024).

As explained in the last section, maintaining stable blood sugar is crucial for the ongoing production of T3, as well as for brain and nerve function (Thyroid Patient Advocacy, 2024; Open Oregon, 2020d).

Hypoglycemia (low blood sugar) can lead to feelings of confusion, shakiness, and irritability, as the brain lacks sufficient glucose. If left unaddressed, it can escalate to seizures and potentially coma, highlighting the importance of the body's mechanisms to preserve blood glucose balance (Open Oregon, 2020e).

When blood sugar levels drop, the body must activate its stress hormones, adrenaline, and cortisol, to raise blood glucose back to normal (Peat R., Glycemia, starch, and sugar in context, 2009c), see Figure 3.4.

Glucose is released from the glycogen stores:

Adrenaline will make the liver release glucose from its glycogen stores, this will provide glucose to maintain brain, nerve, and T3 production for some time (Thyroid Patient Advocacy, 2024; Functional Performance Systems, 2024a).

Typically, a healthy person who has been consuming carbohydrates will have enough glycogen to sustain blood glucose levels for about 24 hours of fasting (Open Oregon, 2020d).

However, many individuals with hypothyroidism may struggle to maintain adequate glycogen stores, and for some people there is only glucose in the liver for a few hours of fasting, making them more susceptible to low blood sugar episodes (Peat R., Nutrition for Women: 100 Short Articles, 2001d, p. 33; Peat R., Glycemia, starch, and sugar in context, 2009c).

The body makes new glucose and ketones:

When the glycogen is depleted, the stress hormones make the body turn protein into glucose and fats into ketones. This adaptation helps ensure that vital functions can continue even under conditions of nutrient scarcity (Open Oregon, 2020e).

Proteins can be turned into glucose:

Cortisol triggers the conversion of protein (amino acids) into glucose through a process known as gluconeogenesis. The protein can come from your diet or muscle tissues (Open Oregon, 2020e). If the diet is deficient in protein, cortisol will facilitate the breakdown of muscles to provide amino acids for the synthesis of glucose (Peat R., Glycemia, starch, and sugar in context, 2009c; Thyroid Patient Advocacy, 2024).

It's crucial to recognize that muscle protein is particularly rich in the amino acids, tryptophan and cysteine. When these amino acids are released from our tissues, they exhibit significant anti-metabolic effects (Functional Performance Systems, 2024a; Thyroid Patient Advocacy, 2024).

Fat can be converted to ketones:

Fats cannot be turned into glucose; however, adrenalin will mobilize fatty acids from the body's fat stores. The free fatty acids can be turned into ketone bodies, which are compounds the brain can use for energy in the absence of glucose (Peat R., Glycemia, starch, and sugar in context, 2009c; Open Oregon, 2020e).

If you have been eating unsaturated fats in the past years, these are stored in your fat tissues and their release to the bloodstream will significantly inhibit your metabolic rate (Peat R., Glycemia, starch, and sugar in context, 2009c; Functional Performance Systems, 2024a).

Stress hormones directly inhibit metabolism:

In addition, the stress hormones themselves directly impair metabolic function. Cortisol and adrenaline inhibit the conversion of T4 to T3 (Peat R., TSH, temperature, pulse rate, and other indicators in hypothyroidism, 2008a, p. 3).

Additionally, adrenaline increases the production of reverse T3 (rT3), an inactive form of T3 that interferes with the functionality of T3 (Peat R., Nutrition for Women: 100 Short Articles, 2001d, p. 20; Peat R., TSH, temperature, pulse rate, and other indicators in hypothyroidism, 2008a).

For further details on how stress and rT3 impact metabolism, I recommend consulting my second book in my "Healing Metabolism" book series" titled "Test Your Thyroid Function".

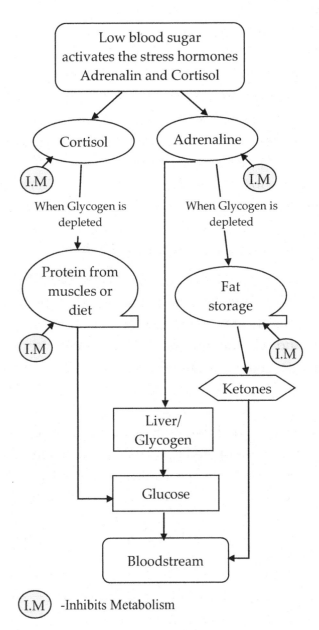

Figure. 3.4: *When blood sugar levels drop, the stress hormones adrenaline and cortisol are released. Adrenaline first prompts the liver to release glucose from its glycogen stores. Once these stores are depleted, cortisol converts proteins (amino acids) into glucose. Additionally, adrenaline transforms fat into ketones, offering the brain an alternative energy source to glucose. Released fatty acids and amino acids can inhibit metabolism. Furthermore, both adrenaline and cortisol directly inhibit metabolism.*

The problem with low carbohydrate diets:

When a person is fasting or eats a very low-carbohydrate diet, like a ketogenic diet (which mainly consists of proteins and fats) the blood sugar drops, and all the mechanisms described above come into play (Khan Academy, 2024; Open Oregon, 2020e).

Dr. Ray Peat argued that both fasting and ketogenic diets should be avoided because they can negatively impact metabolic rate and lead to persistently high levels of cortisol. High cortisol levels can result in muscle wasting and premature aging, as cortisol is a catabolic hormone that breaks down tissues (Ryan Heeney, 2018).

Dr. Peat strongly advised against low-carbohydrate diets and recommended consuming plenty of healthy carbohydrates daily. He defined healthy carbohydrates as those that stabilize blood sugar. Additionally, it's crucial to consider the vitamin and mineral content and the effects on digestion when selecting carbohydrates (Thyroid Patient Advocacy, 2024).

In the following sections, I will explore different types of carbohydrates and discuss their impact on blood sugar, metabolic performance, and digestive health.

Key Points – Low Blood Sugar:

Low blood sugar inhibits the liver enzyme responsible for converting T4 to T3.

Low blood sugar increases the levels of stress hormones adrenaline and cortisol.

Adrenaline and cortisol directly inhibit the conversion of T4 to T3.

Adrenaline increases the production of rT3, which blocks the function of the active thyroid hormone T3.

Adrenaline releases free fatty acids from fat stores; if these are unsaturated, they will inhibit the metabolic rate.

Cortisol promotes the degradation of muscle tissue, leading to the release of anti-metabolic amino acids.

Eating plenty of healthy carbohydrates throughout the day is important for stabilizing blood sugar and metabolism.

Fasting and low carbohydrate diets should be avoided.

The Issues with Starches

Rice, bread, pasta, cereal, and similar foods are rich in starch, which is composed of long chains of glucose molecules linked together (Open Oregon, 2020b; Open Oregon, 2020d).

While starchy foods are often perceived as healthier than sugar, they can disrupt blood sugar levels, potentially impairing the metabolic rate. Furthermore, starches are known to promote fat storage (Peat R., Glycemia, starch, and sugar in context, 2009c; Harvard T.H. Chan, 2024).

Starches overstimulate insulin secretion:

Starch is rapidly digested and broken down into glucose that is quickly absorbed into the bloodstream (Harvard T.H. Chan, 2024).

The glycemic index ranks foods according to their ability to raise blood sugar and starches have a very high glycemic index (Healthline, 2023; Peat R., Glycemia, starch, and sugar in context, 2009c).

The spike in blood sugar that follows the consumption of a starchy meal triggers a massive release of insulin. Insulin, a hormone produced by the pancreas, enables cells to take up glucose from the bloodstream (Peat R., Glycemia, starch, and sugar in context, 2009c).

Starches lower blood sugar:

The massive secretion of insulin that follows a high-starch meal can lower blood sugar below normal levels (Peat R., Glycemia, starch, and sugar in context, 2009c). Low blood sugar directly inhibits the conversion of T4 to the active thyroid hormone T3. Additionally, low blood sugar triggers stress responses that further impair the metabolic rate. Starches promote obesity:

Eating starch raises insulin levels and lowers blood sugar, which in turn stimulates appetite and leads to increased food intake. Additionally, the massive release of insulin following a high-starch meal promotes the conversion of glucose into fat. Dr. Ray Peat emphasized that a high-starch diet promotes obesity (Peat R., Glycemia, starch, and sugar in context, 2009c).

Can I have starches on the "Ray Peat diet":

In many Western countries, diets heavily rely on starches: cereal for breakfast, bread for lunch, and pasta or rice for dinner.

Ray Peat consistently cautioned against making starches the foundation of one's diet. However, this does not imply that all starches should be eliminated. I have observed that entirely removing starches from the diet can lead to feelings of deprivation in many individuals.

Nevertheless, consuming large amounts of starches alone is discouraged (Peat R., Glycemia, starch, and sugar in context, 2009c). Yet, some starches can be moderately incorporated into your diet when appropriately combined with other foods.

Safe starches:

Dr. Ray Peat particularly favored starches from well-cooked potatoes and tortillas made from lime-treated corn flour (Masa Harina). He considered these safe starches that can be eaten in abundance. Tortillas made from lime-treated corn are also a great substitute for bread (#55: Bioenergetic Nutrition Basics I, 2021).

How to make your starches less problematic:

Starches become much less problematic when consumed with sources of fructose, such as orange juice, and saturated fats like cheese, butter, or coconut oil (Ray Peat Clips, 2016n).

Consuming saturated fats with your starches slows their absorption from the intestine, which mitigates their tendency to spike blood glucose (Ray Peat Clips, 2016v; Food Research International, 2021). Fructose helps counteract the significant insulin spike that starches typically cause (Peat R., Glycemia, starch, and sugar in context, 2009c), a topic which will be discussed further in the following section.

The Benefits of Fructose

Sucrose, as mentioned, is a disaccharide found in fruits, honey, and table sugar, composed of 50% glucose and 50% fructose (Open Oregon, 2020d).

While table sugar consists purely of sucrose, fruits and honey also contain free monosaccharides in the form of glucose and fructose. Typically, the ratio of fructose to glucose in fruits and honey is approximately 50% of each (Medical News Today, 2024).

In contrast, starch is the only naturally occurring carbohydrate that consists entirely of glucose (Open Oregon, 2020d).

Fructose offers significant health benefits, causing sugar, fruit, and honey to behave very differently in the body compared to starch (Ray Peat Clips, 2010c; Peat R., Glycemia, starch, and sugar in context, 2009c).

Fructose stabilizes blood sugar:

Fructose is slowly converted into glucose, which means it does not cause a rapid increase in blood glucose levels like starches do. In other words, fructose has a low glycemic index and does not excessively stimulate insulin secretion (Open Oregon, 2020c; Ray Peat Clips, 2016r; Another School of Thought Radio, 2011).

Fructose even helps prevent the massive secretion of insulin induced by glucose (Peat R., Glycemia, starch, and sugar in context, 2009c). Fructose also blocks insulin's tendency to promote obesity (Ray Peat Clips, 2016s).

In addition, fructose enhances the liver's capacity to store glycogen and thus helps maintain steady blood sugar levels (Another School of Thought Radio, 2011).

Fructose stimulates metabolism:

Fructose stimulates the metabolic rate in several ways, activating various components of the thyroid system, including the production of T3 (Ray Peat Clips, 2016n; Ray Peat clips, 2016q).

Including fructose as part of a balanced diet can significantly improve the metabolic rate. It almost acts like the active thyroid hormone T3, catalyzing the body's ability to burn calories and convert glucose into biological energy (ATP) (Another School of Thought Radio, 2011).

Dr. Ray Peat emphasized that the presence of fructose in sugar, honey, and fruits helps stabilize blood sugar, improve metabolism, and prevent obesity, whereas starches (pure glucose), do the opposite (Peat R., Glycemia, starch, and sugar in context, 2009c).

Key Points – Carbohydrates & Blood sugar:

Starch is 100% glucose. Starch has a high glycemic index, leading to a spike in blood sugar and subsequent overstimulation of insulin secretion.

High insulin lowers blood sugar, which impairs metabolism and promotes overeating. High insulin stimulates fat synthesis and promotes obesity.

Fruit, honey, and sugar contain 50% glucose and 50% fructose. Since fructose is slowly converted into glucose, fruit, honey, and sugar don't spike blood sugar.

Fructose stabilizes blood sugar and supports thyroid function. Fructose prevents the overstimulation of insulin and blocks insulin's tendency to create obesity.

Healthy carbohydrates come from sweet fruits, honey, sugar, and safe starches such as potatoes and tortillas.

Starches become less problematic if they are eaten with saturated fats and fructose (fruit).

I Thought Sugar was Harmful

Many health professionals and doctors link sugar consumption to obesity, type 2 diabetes, and fungal overgrowth, among other health issues. However, Dr. Ray Peat did not share these concerns.

Sugar does not promote obesity:

As described in the previous section, excessive insulin secretion promotes obesity. The fructose found in sugar, honey, and fruit prevents excessive insulin secretion and even blocks insulin's tendency to promote obesity. Additionally, fructose supports a high metabolic rate, thereby increasing calorie burn (Peat R., Glycemia, starch, and sugar in context, 2009c; Peat R., Generative Energy, 2001a, pp. 73-74).

Sugar does not cause type 2 diabetes:

Type 2 diabetes is characterized by insulin resistance, where cells are unable to absorb glucose from the bloodstream. As a result, any cellular function requiring glucose is impaired (Peat R., Glucose and sucrose for diabetes, 2016a). Dr. Ray Peat emphasized that the problem in diabetes is the lack of glucose within the cells, not its excess in the bloodstream (Another School of Thought Radio,

2011; Peat R., Glucose and sucrose for diabetes, 2016a).

According to Dr. Peat, it is well established that polyunsaturated fats (PUFAs), rather than sugars, are responsible for the insulin resistance characteristic of type 2 diabetes (Peat R., Glucose and sucrose for diabetes, 2016a; Another School of Thought Radio, 2011).

Yeast infection management:

In cases of intestinal yeast (candida) overgrowth, the common advice is to avoid sugars, including fruits. However, completely depriving yeast of sugar can be counterproductive, as the yeast may become invasive.

When starved of sugar, yeast develops filaments that can penetrate intestinal tissues in search of sugar. Therefore, consuming sugar in moderation acts defensively by preventing the yeast from becoming invasive (Another School of Thought Radio, 2011).

The most effective way to combat an intestinal yeast infection is to maintain a high metabolic rate and incorporate Dr. Ray Peat's carrot salad into your daily diet. This approach helps suppress the growth of yeast and supports overall intestinal health (Another School of Thought Radio, 2011). You will learn about the benefits of raw carrots and how to make Dr. Ray Peat's famous carrot salad later in this chapter.

Key Points – Sugar & Health Issues:

Sugar does not cause type 2 diabetes. Instead, PUFAs are the cause of this condition.

Sugar eaten in moderation does not promote obesity. Instead, a diet high in PUFAs and starches promotes this condition.

Sugar does not have to be avoided in yeast infections.

Moderate use of normal white sugar and honey can be part of a healthy diet.

Benedicte Mai Lerche MSc PhD

Harmful Fibers & Whole Grains

We often hear that fiber is healthy and beneficial for our digestive system. In the following, I will outline Dr. Ray Peat's perspective on fiber and explain why most fiber-rich foods should be avoided.

Dietary fibers are found in whole grains, seeds, nuts, legumes, crisp and unripe fruits, undercooked vegetables, raw salads, and similar foods (Ray Peat Clips, 2016o; Open Oregon, 2020d).

Whole-grain versions of bread, pasta, and rice are often recommended as healthier options than their refined counterparts. Indeed, whole-grain products provide slightly more vitamins and minerals. (Ray Peat Clips, 2016o). However, whole grains contain both the germ and the bran, which are rich in polyunsaturated fats (PUFAs) and dietary fibers, respectively (Harvard T.H. Chan, 2024)

Fiber and gut health:

As mentioned at the beginning of this chapter, fibers are long chains of glucose, but human digestive enzymes cannot break them down, so we do not get nutritional value from consuming fibers. Consequently, these dietary fibers travel to the large intestine, where they can become food for resident bacteria through fermentation. This fermentation process generates gas, which explains why consuming a fibrous meal can cause bloating and flatulence (Open Oregon, 2020c).

While many nutritionists advocate for feeding gut bacteria with dietary fiber, Dr. Ray Peat highlighted concerns that an overgrowth of intestinal bacteria can cause significant health problems (Ray Peat Clips, 2016p).

Gut bacteria constantly produce endotoxins, which don't cause any health issues under normal circumstances. However, feeding the gut bacteria with dietary fibers could potentially lead to bacterial overgrowth, resulting in the production of excessive amounts of endotoxins (Ray Peat clips, 2016t). (Erlanson-Albertsson C, 2021; Ray Peat clips, 2009; Ray Peat clips, 2016t)

Endotoxins irritate the intestine, triggering the production of inflammatory mediators like nitric oxide (Ray Peat Clips, 2016l; Ray Peat Clips, 2016y). This inflammation can become severe enough to cause the intestine to become "leaky," allowing bacteria, endotoxins, nitric oxide, and other inflammatory mediators to enter the bloodstream, potentially leading to systemic inflammation (Ray Peat Clips, 2016y). Additionally, nitric oxide significantly impairs metabolism (Ray Peat Clips, 2016y; KMUD, 2015).

Dr. Ray Peat emphasized that intestinal inflammation is associated with a slow metabolic rate, obesity, and chronic fatigue. Consequently, he recommended avoiding fiber-rich foods to prevent bacterial overgrowth in the gut (KMUD, 2015).

How to avoid dietary fibers:

Many fiber-rich foods are already excluded from the Ray Peat diet due to other components such as phytoestrogens in legumes and PUFAs in nuts, seeds, and grains.

Dr. Ray Peat emphasized that if you choose to include bread, pasta, and rice in your diet, it is preferable to consume refined products, as they have had both the germ and bran removed. This means that white rice, bread, and pasta do not contain PUFAs or dietary fibers (Harward T. H. Chan , 2024).

Additionally, Dr. Ray Peat recommended avoiding raw salads, undercooked vegetables, and crisp fruits. He explained that cooking these fiber-rich foods breaks down their fibers, making them more digestible (Ray Peat clips, 2016t).

Therefore, it is advisable to cook your vegetables thoroughly. Dr. Peat was especially fond of well-cooked potatoes.

Instead of consuming crisp fruits like apples and pears, Dr. Peat advised cooking them into compotes or sauces (Ray Peat clips, 2016t).

Furthermore, eating saturated fats (such as butter, coconut oil, or wiped cream) with these well-cooked, fiber-rich foods can help prevent the overgrowth of gut bacteria (Ray Peat Clips, 2016ø).

It is important to mention that carrots are the only vegetable Dr. Ray Peat consistently advised eating raw. Raw carrots hold a special place in the "Ray Peat diet" framework, which is the topic of the next section.

Beneficial Antimicrobial Fibers

In the previous section, I highlighted how dietary fiber can feed gut bacteria, potentially causing bacterial overgrowth and intestinal inflammation. However, this doesn't mean that all fibers should be avoided. Dr. Ray Peat emphasized the importance of incorporating what he called antimicrobial fibers into the daily diet.

Antimicrobial fibers are found in raw carrots and cooked bamboo shoots. These vegetables, which grow in moist and dark underground conditions, have developed antimicrobial substances that protect them from germs and microbes (Ray Peat Clips, 2016m; KMUD: Bowel Endotoxin, 2009).

The antimicrobial substances in raw carrots and cooked bamboo shoots prevent these fibers from becoming food for bacteria in the intestine. This allows us to benefit from their fiber content without promoting bacterial growth (Ray Peat Clips, 2016m).

In the gut, these antimicrobial substances act like natural antibiotics, inhibiting the overgrowth of bacteria and fungi (Candida) (Ray Peat Clips, 2016m).

Additionally, these fibers help with bowel movements and bind to endotoxins and estrogen, assisting the body in eliminating these harmful compounds (Ray Peat Clips, 2016m).

Several individuals have reported improvements in symptoms of PMS, allergies, and headaches due to daily consumption of antimicrobial fibers (Peat R., From PMS to Menopause: Female Hormones in Context, 2001b, p. 189).

Dr. Ray Peat has noted that daily consumption of either raw carrots or cooked bamboo shoots can significantly improve gut health and hormonal balance (Eluv Radio: Stress and Trauma, 2014c).

Regular consumption of antimicrobial fibers lowers estrogen and cortisol levels and increases progesterone levels. These changes support your metabolism, as estrogen and cortisol inhibit the metabolic rate, while progesterone enhances it (Peat R., From PMS to Menopause: Female Hormones in Context, 2001b, p. 93).

How to eat your bamboo shoots:

You'll often find canned bamboo shoots in supermarkets, which are perfectly fine to use. After boiling your bamboo shoots, they can be added to any dish you like.

How to eat your carrots:

Carrots should always be eaten raw to preserve their antimicrobial fibers; cooking or juicing them will destroy the fibers and release carotene, which has anti-thyroid effects similar to PUFAs (Ray Peat Clips, 2016z). Dr. Peat recommended eating a large raw carrot daily for its antimicrobial benefits. For an enhanced effect, consider preparing Dr. Ray Peat's famous carrot salad. (Peat R., From PMS to Menopause: Female Hormones in Context, 2001b, pp. 40-41).

Dr. Ray Peat's famous carrot salad:

Dr. Ray Peat's famous carrot salad consists of raw carrots, grated lengthwise to create long fibers. It is served with a dressing made from saturated fats (such as olive oil, coconut oil, or MCT oil), vinegar (free from additives), salt, pepper, and optionally, garlic (Peat R., From PMS to Menopause: Female Hormones in Context, 2001b, p. 189).

The combination of saturated fats and the acetic acid from the vinegar enhances the germicidal effect of the carrot fibers (Peat R., Generative Energy, 2001a,

p. 105; Peat R., From PMS to Menopause: Female Hormones in Context, 2001b, p. 189)

Olive oil can be used alone or mixed with coconut oil, as coconut oil is known to promote thyroid function more than olive oil. MCT oil is also an option, provided you are not allergic to it. For variety, you can add lime juice, meat, cheese, tomatoes, bell peppers, and other ingredients to the salad (Peat R., From PMS to Menopause: Female Hormones in Context, 2001b, p. 189).

When you consume raw carrots or cooked bamboo shoots, the fibers decrease the absorption of other substances eaten at the same time. Therefore, it is advised not to take supplements or medication concurrently with these fibers.

If you choose to eat raw carrots or cooked bamboo shoots with your meals, they will reduce the amount of food absorbed, thereby aiding in weight loss (Functional Performance Systems, 2024b).

Key Points – Dietary Fibers:

Dietary fibers can feed gut bacteria and cause intestinal inflammation.

Fiber-rich foods such as whole grains, legumes, nuts, seeds, raw salads, raw vegetables, and crisp fruits should be avoided.

It is better to eat refined rice, bread, and pasta than their whole grain versions.

Vegetables and crisp fruits should be thoroughly cooked and eaten with saturated fats.

Antimicrobial fibers from either raw carrots or cooked bamboo shoots should be incorporated into the daily diet.

You can choose to eat one or two raw carrots per day or optimize the antimicrobial effect by making Dr. Ray Peat's famous carrot salad.

Benedicte Mai Lerche MSc PhD

Bread on the Ray Peat Diet

As discussed throughout this chapter, starches can disrupt blood sugar levels and contribute to obesity.

However, if avoiding bread entirely proves too challenging, consider opting for sourdough bread made from refined wheat flour that has been slowly raised for at least 9 hours. Refined wheat flour is devoid of the germ and bran, which eliminates PUFAs and fibers (Harward T. H. Chan , 2024).

The extended, gradual rising period allows for the breakdown of starch and gluten in the wheat flour, resulting in bread that is more nutritious and easier to digest. Those with gluten sensitivity often find they can tolerate "slow-risen" sourdough bread without experiencing adverse symptoms (Nashoba Brook Bakery Bread , 2024; Jodellefit, Dr. Ray Peat - Liver Health, Milk, Alcohol, and More Listener Q&A, 2021).

The glycemic index of "slow-risen" sourdough bread is much lower than that of "quick-rise" bread, such as those typically found at commercial bakeries or supermarkets (Nashoba Brook Bakery Bread , 2024).

Although slowly raised sourdough bread made from refined wheat flour is nutritionally superior to other bread types, it remains a starch that can stimulate appetite and activate fat synthesis. Conversely, the same caloric intake from fruit would be less fattening, helping to maintain steadier blood sugar levels and potentially improving your metabolic rate (Expulsia, 2024c).

Another potentially superior substitute for commercial quick-risen bread is tortillas made from lime-treated corn flour (Masa Harina). These tortillas are a safe type of starch that can be consumed in abundance without any problems (#55: Bioenergetic Nutrition Basics I, 2021). Additionally, Masa Harina tortillas are rich in calcium, which has numerous health benefits—a topic that will be discussed in the next chapter.

Key Points – Two Substitutes for Bread:

Sourdough bread made from refined wheat flour that has been slowly raised for at least 9 hours.

Tortillas made from lime-treated corn flour (Masa Harina), fried in coconut oil.

Fruit, Honey, and Sugar

Due to the widespread advice to reduce sugar intake, many people strive to avoid sugar, honey, and sometimes even sweet fruits and fruit juices.

Dr. Ray Peat offered an alternative perspective. His dietary advice includes minimizing starches from bread, pasta rice cereal, etc, and instead obtaining healthy carbohydrates primarily from ripe, low-starchy fruits. According to Dr. Peat, even honey and white sugar have their place in a balanced diet (Another School of Thought Radio, 2011; Peat R., Glycemia, starch, and sugar in context, 2009c).

As previously explained, the fructose in sweet, low-starch fruits, white sugar, and honey makes these simple carbohydrates healthier than starches. Unlike starches, which can overstimulate insulin secretion, these simple sugars help stabilize blood sugar and promote metabolism (Peat R., Glycemia, starch, and sugar in context, 2009c).

Minerals in fruits:

In addition to fructose, fruits provide essential minerals like potassium and magnesium, which also help stabilize blood sugar levels. In contrast, white sugar contains no minerals, and honey only contains small amounts. This means that fruits offer better blood sugar-stabilizing effects compared to honey and white sugar (Another School of Thought Radio, 2011).

Amount of white sugar and honey:

Dr. Ray Peat's endorsement of sugars primarily refers to those found in fruits. Additionally, his diet supports the moderate use of regular white table sugar and honey (Another School of Thought Radio, 2011).

Brown sugar and dark-colored syrups:

Brown sugar and dark-colored syrups, such as molasses, maple syrup, and agave syrup, contain more minerals than white sugar. However, Dr. Ray Peat explained that these sugars also contain impurities that can potentially cause allergies (Another School of Thought Radio, 2011; Ray Peat KMUD Food Additives Full Interview, 2009g; Peat R., From PMS to Menopause: Female Hormones in Context, 2001b, p. 189).

Best fruits:

Dr. Ray Peat recommended consuming low-starch ripe fruits, which are rich in beneficial sugars and low in indigestible fibers. He often mentioned papayas, melons, grapes, peaches, guavas, and citrus fruits as particularly beneficial.

Dr. Peat was very fond of citrus fruits, as they are rich in good sugars, minerals, and naringenin, which has anti-estrogenic properties. However, he advised against consuming grapefruits because they contain a chemical that inhibits a liver enzyme necessary for detoxifying estrogen (Another School of Thought Radio, 2011).

Orange juice:

Dr. Ray Peat drank large amounts of pulp-free orange juice daily, explaining that pulp-free is best because the pulp (fiber) can feed gut bacteria, potentially leading to their overgrowth. Freshly pressed orange juice from sweet oranges is ideal, but even store-bought pasteurized pulp-free orange juice can significantly support your metabolism. Dr. Peat also noted that orange juice from concentrate offers many health benefits, emphasizing that one shouldn't refrain from consuming orange juice simply because the finest quality is not available

(#55: Bioenergetic Nutrition Basics I, 2021; Another School of Thought Radio, 2011).

Cooking crisp fruits:

Crisp fruits such as apples and pears should be avoided due to their high fiber content, which can lead to gut bacterial overgrowth. Cooking crisp fruits into compotes or sauces and pairing them with saturated fats like whipped cream provides a delicious and healthy dessert.

Indulging in sweets:

Dr. Peat did not object to occasionally indulging in sweets. Consuming a Coca-Cola, a piece of high-quality chocolate, a cup of homemade hot chocolate (made from milk, sugar, and cacao powder), or some gummy bears made from sugar, gelatin, and fruit concentrate can be acceptable (Another School of Thought Radio, 2011)

It is crucial to note that many store-bought sweets are made with glucose syrup instead of sugar. Like starch, glucose syrup overstimulates insulin production, disrupts blood sugar levels, and promotes obesity.

Sugar from dairy products:

Additionally, dairy products such as milk, cheese, and Greek yogurt contain lactose (milk sugar), which Dr. Ray Peat considered a very healthy form of carbohydrate (Another School of Thought Radio, 2011).

Pure fructose powder:

Pure fructose powder, which is 100% fructose, is often available in supermarkets, health food stores, and online. Dr. Ray Peat explained that pure fructose powder can be particularly helpful for people with diabetes and hypoglycemia (low blood sugar), as it is especially good at stabilizing blood sugar levels (Another School of Thought Radio, 2011).

You can use fructose powder to sweeten tea, coffee, Greek yogurt, or other foods. There aren't any strict guidelines on how much fructose powder to use. If you incorporate something like 3-4 tablespoons of fructose powder into your daily diet, reducing your intake of other sugars is recommended to prevent exceeding your daily caloric needs.

It is important to note that some may experience allergic reactions to fructose powder, which might be linked to its manufacturing process (Another School of Thought Radio, 2011)

Previously, I described the negative consequences of eating starches, including their ability to lower blood sugar and promote obesity. If you eat some sweet fruit or fructose powder before or together with a starchy meal such as bread, pasta, or rice, you can create a better balance between glucose and fructose, thus preventing the spike in blood glucose and the overstimulation of insulin.

Artificial Sweeteners:

Most artificial sweeteners are not inherently dangerous, but they should be avoided because they might confuse the sugar metabolism, leading to stress-related problems. In addition, artificial sweeteners are very bad for losing weight, as their sweet taste activates the appetite.

Key Points – Fruit, Honey, and Sugar:

Healthy carbohydrates primarily come from low-starch sweet ripe fruits, milk products, and moderate amounts of honey, white table sugar as well as fructose powder.

Dr. Ray Peat was especially fond of papayas, melons, grapes, peaches, guavas, and citrus fruits.

It is advisable to drink pulp-free orange juice. It is important to avoid grapefruits as they can increase estrogen levels.

White sugar is preferred over brown sugar and dark-colored syrups.

Artificial sweeteners should be avoided.

Benedicte Mai Lerche MSc PhD

Advice on Vegetables

Many people like to include vegetables in their diets. Choosing the safest ones requires considering several factors, which is the topic of this section.

Avoid raw vegetables from the cabbage family:

Ray Peat generally advised against consuming undercooked vegetables due to their fiber content. Additionally, it is important to remember that raw vegetables from the cabbage family inhibit thyroid function (Peat R., From PMS to Menopause: Female Hormones in Context, 2001b, p. 78).

The cabbage family of vegetables, also known as Brassicaceae or Cruciferae includes, among others, broccoli, Brussels sprouts, cabbage, Napa cabbage, cauliflower, Chinese broccoli, collards, daikon, kale, kohlrabi, mustard greens, mustard seeds, rutabaga, turnip, radish, Bok choy, watercress, and wasabi. These vegetables contain compounds known as goitrogens (Peat R., From PMS to Menopause: Female Hormones in Context, 2001b, p. 78; Everyday Health, 2018).

Goitrogens can negatively impact thyroid health by interfering with the thyroid gland's ability to absorb iodine, which is crucial for the synthesis of thyroid hormones (Cleveland Clinic, 2019).

Most goitrogens are neutralized by thorough cooking. Therefore, if you choose to consume vegetables from the cabbage family, it is crucial to boil them thoroughly (Rogers K., 2024).

Plants contain toxins (anti-nutrients):

Plants contain defensive toxic chemicals, primarily concentrated in their seeds and their above-ground parts, meaning leaves and stems (Another School of Thought Radio, 2011). These toxic chemicals serve to discourage insects, birds, and grazing animals (Peat R., Vegetables, etc.—Who Defines Food?, 2006c).

Plant toxins are often referred to as anti-nutrients as they can interfere with human digestive enzymes, hinder the absorption of vitamins and minerals, and disrupt various metabolic processes (Peat R., Vegetables, etc.—Who Defines Food?, 2006c; Open Biotechnology Journal, 2019).

Dr. Ray Peat often mentioned leafy green vegetables as good sources of calcium and other important minerals and emphasized that they can be consumed safely if they are cooked thoroughly to destroy their anti-nutrients (Eluv Radio: Stress and Trauma, 2014a).

He also pointed out that fruits and root vegetables tend to offer high concentrations of important nutrients while containing low levels of toxic substances (Peat R., Vegetables, etc.—Who Defines Food?, 2006c).

Root vegetables:

The underground parts of plants, like roots and tubers, are less accessible to grazing animals and insects and therefore contain fewer digestive inhibitors compared to the above-ground parts. Instead, roots and tubers contain chemicals that inhibit microorganisms (Peat R., Vegetables, etc.—Who Defines Food?, 2006c).

Dr. Ray Peat recommended a variety of root vegetables, with a particular preference for white potatoes. Potatoes not only provide carbohydrates but also contain protein and keto acids, which will be discussed further in the next chapter (Another School of Thought Radio, 2011).

It is crucial to boil all your root vegetables thoroughly and consume them with ample saturated fats. Carrots are, as explained, the only exception, as cooking or juicing the carrots releases their carotene, which possesses anti-thyroid properties.

Fruit–like vegetables:

Beyond root vegetables, Dr. Peat endorses several low-starchy vegetables that are technically fruits. He frequently highlighted small summer squashes (zucchini) as particularly beneficial (Another School of Thought Radio, 2011).

Other favorable low-starch fruit-like vegetables include tomatoes, cucumbers, sweet peppers, olives, and eggplants (aubergines) (Breyer, 2019).

It's important to note that while pumpkins and winter squashes are categorized as fruits, those with orange flesh are high in carotene, which has anti-thyroid effects (Ray Peat clips, 2017).

Tomatoes, cucumbers, sweet peppers, and olives are ideal for consuming raw and make excellent bases for salads. Enhancing their flavors can easily be achieved with a dressing composed of olive oil, vinegar, salt, pepper, and garlic.

Meanwhile, summer squashes and eggplants, along with non-orange-fleshed pumpkins and winter squashes, should be cooked and eaten with butter or coconut oil.

Key Points – Advice on vegstables:

Raw vegetables contain toxic compounds called anti-nutrient.

Raw vegetables from the cabbage family contain goitrogens that inhibit thyroid function.

Generally it is important to avoid raw and undercooked vegetables. Cooking your vegetables breaks down their fibers and destroys most of the problematic toxins and goitrogens.

The safest vegetables are root vegstables and vegetables that are technically fruits.

Low-starch fruit-like vegetables such as tomatoes, cucumbers, sweet peppers, and olives are ideal for consuming raw.

Starchy root vegetables like white potatoes and fruit-like vegetables such as summer squashes, and eggplants, pumpkins and winter squashes, should be cooked and eaten with butter or coconut oil.

List of Bad Carbohydrates

Avoid the following carbohydrates:

- Whole grains seeds and nuts
- Raw salads and undercooked vegetables
- Raw crisp fruits like apples and pears
- Grapefruits
- Raw vegetables from the cabbage family
- Sweet potatoes
- Cooked or juiced carrots
- Orange flesh pumpkins and winter squashes
- Brown sugar and dark-colored syrups.
- Artificial sweeteners

Limit starches:

- Bread,
- Pasta
- Rice
- Cereal etc.

Benedicte Mai Lerche MSc PhD

List of Good Carbohydrates

Sugars:

- White table sugar
- Honey
- Pure fructose powder
- Dairy products (lactose)

Examples of good low-starch sweet fruits:

- Orange juice (without pulp)
- Lemon juice (without pulp)
- Watermelon and other melons
- Cherries
- Apricots
- Dads/raisins/figs (fresh or dried)
- Berries
- Grapes and grape juice
- Peaches and nectarines
- Papaya
- Guava
- Pawpaw
- Lychee (canned is OK)
- Cooked apples (apple sauce)
- Cooked pears (fruit compote)

Crisp fruits, such as apples and pears, should be cooked and consumed with saturated fats like homemade ice cream, whipped cream, or Greek yogurt. Some fruits, such as applesauce and lychees, can be found canned, which is a good option when fresh fruits are not available.

Good vegetables:

The best vegetables are root vegetables and those vegetables that are technically fruits. Vegetables marked with a star (*) can be eaten raw. Otherwise, the listed vegetables should be thoroughly cooked and consumed with butter or coconut oil.

Examples of good root vegetables:

- White potatoes
- Celery root
- Parsley root
- Leeks
- Jerusalem artichokes
- Onions, spring onions and garlic*
- Sugar beets
- Turmeric
- Ginger

Examples of good fruit-like vegetables:

- Sommer squashes
- Eggplants
- Cucumber*
- Tomatoes*
- Chili peppers*
- Bell peppers/sweet peppers*
- Olives*

Important antimicrobial fibers:

- Raw carrots* (never cook or juice your carrots)
- Cooked Bamboo shots.

The fibers from raw carrots and cooked bamboo shoots are important for your intestinal health, and it is recommended to include either of these fibers in your daily diet.

Good alternatives to commercial bread:

- Tortillas made from lime-treated corn flour
- Sourdough bread, made from refined wheat flour (slow-risen for more than 9 hours)

Chapter 4: Proteins

Benedicte Mai Lerche MSc PhD

How Protein Affects Metabolism

Dr. Ray Peat highlighted the critical importance of consuming at least 100 grams (3½ ounces) of high-quality protein daily, noting that insufficient protein intake can drastically impair your metabolic rate and overall health (Ray Peat Clips, 2016h; Peat R., Nutrition for Women: 100 Short Articles, 2001d, p. 96; Peat R., Generative Energy, 2001a, pp. 73-74; #55: Bioenergetic Nutrition Basics I, 2021).

Dr. Ray Peat explained that about 100 grams of protein daily is needed for both men and women to perform normal office work, with the protein requirement increasing with more physical activity (Peat R., Gelatin, stress, longevity, 2004). In Table 3.1, you can see the protein content of some foods that are also part of the "Ray Peat diet".

Dr. Peat further emphasized that many people who don't respond to their thyroid medication are simply not consuming enough high-quality protein (Thyroid Patient Advocacy, 2024).

The liver, which plays a pivotal role in converting T4 into the active thyroid hormone T3, requires high-quality protein for optimal function. This underscores the necessity of ensuring adequate protein intake to facilitate the production of T3 (Peat R., Generative Energy, 2001a, pp. 73-74).

The liver is also key in detoxification and crucial for removing estrogen and endotoxins. Therefore, a lack of dietary protein can also result in estrogen dominance and inflammation (Peat R., Natural estrogens, 2008b; Peat R., Vegetables, etc. —Who Defines Food?, 2006c).

In the current health and environmental discourse, vegetable protein sources are often highlighted as beneficial (Medical News Today, 2023a); however, Dr. Ray Peat identified several issues with obtaining protein from foods such as beans, lentils, nuts, seeds, and soy products (Peat R., From PMS to Menopause: Female Hormones in Context, 2001b, pp. 19-20; Peat R., Nutrition for Women: 100 Short Articles, 2001d, p. 17). While he did recommend a few vegetable sources of protein, his general recommendation leaned towards high-quality protein from animal-based foods such as milk, cheese, eggs, shellfish, white fish, beef, lamb, and gelatine (Peat R., Nutrition for Women: 100 Short Articles, 2001d).

Choosing the right animal protein sources involves recognizing that non-ruminant meats, like pork and poultry, typically contain significant amounts of polyunsaturated fats (PUFAs), a trait shared with oily fish. Furthermore, muscle meats should be limited as they are high in amino acids that can dampen metabolism (Peat R., Nutrition for Women: 100 Short Articles, 2001d, p. 81). Conversely, milk, eggs, shellfish, and liver are valuable for their rich content of vital minerals and vitamins.

This chapter will delve into the subject of identifying the best sources of both vegetable and animal proteins, making it easier for you to select foods rich in high-quality protein that supports your metabolism. To understand the different aspects of proteins it is necessary to comprehend the structure of proteins, which is the focus of the next section.

High-Quality Protein Food list	
Food	**Protein content per 100g of food**
Gelatin	87 g
Cow and Calf	20-24 g
Calf liver	19 g
Goat	27 g
Sheep and Lamb	20 g
Deer	23 g
Shrimp	24 g
Crab	19 g
Lobster	19 g
Clam and Mussel	25 g
Cod	18 g
Eggs	13 g
Low-fat milk	3.4 g
Greek Yoghurt	10 g
Cheese	25 g
Potatoes	3.4 g
Mushrooms	3.4 g

Table 3.1: Table showing the approximate protein content in some protein-rich foods, that are part of the "Ray Peat diet". 1 oz ≃28g and 100g≃3.5 oz (Healthbeet.org, 2024; Johns Hopkins medicine, 2024).

The Structure of Proteins

Proteins also called polypeptides are large molecules made up of amino acids, which are referred to as the building blocks of proteins (Open Oregon Educational Science, 2020a).

In proteins 50 or more amino acids are bound together, just like pearls on a string (Rogers K., 2016; Open Oregon Educational Science, 2020a).

Polypeptide Chain

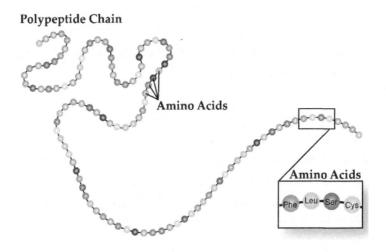

Figure 3.1: Illustration of a polypeptide chain consisting of amino acids linked together like pearls on a string.

There are 20 natural occurring amino acids. You might recognize names like glycine, proline, glutamine, methionine, and others (Koshland, 2014; Open Oregon Educational Science, 2020a).

The human body contains more than 100,000 distinct proteins. This vast array of proteins arises from the virtually limitless combinations of amino acid sequences that can be formed using the 20 natural amino acids (Open Oregon Educational Science, 2020a).

Proteins with similar functions tend to share comparable amino acid compositions and sequences (Koshland, 2014).

In the human body proteins are abundant in muscles, red blood cells, hair, skin, bones, the liver, and various other organs and tissues. It's also crucial to note that all enzymes are proteins, as are many hormones, including insulin (Koshland, 2014). Some proteins, like collagen, are exceptionally large, comprising more than 1,000 amino acids (Open Oregon Educational Science, 2020a). Collagen accounts for about 30% of the body's total protein and is a foundational component of the skin, muscles, bones, tendons, ligaments, and other connective tissues (Cleveland Clinic, 2022c).

The body synthesizes its proteins from amino acids, which it either produces independently or obtains through the diet (Open Oregon Educational Science, 2020a).

There are 11 nonessential amino acids, labeled as such because the body can synthesize them independently. On the other hand, there are 9 essential amino acids that the body cannot produce in sufficient quantities, necessitating their intake through the diet (Open Oregon Educational Science, 2020a). During infancy, periods of growth, and in states of disease, the body might be unable to generate adequate amounts of certain nonessential amino acids. Under these circumstances, an increased dietary intake of these amino acids is needed. Such amino acids are known as conditionally essential amino acids (Open Oregon Educational Science, 2020a).

According to Dr. Ray Peat, three amino acids—tryptophan, methionine, and cysteine—have anti-metabolic properties, and their intake should be limited in adulthood. This subject will be discussed in more detail later in this chapter. In Table 3.2 below you find the 20 natural aminoacids grouped into different categories.

Essential	Nonessential
Histidine	Alanine
Isoleucine	Arginine*
Leucine	Asparagine
Lysine	Aspartic Acid
<u>Methionine</u>	<u>Cysteine*</u>
Phenylalanine	Glutamic Acid
Threonine	Glutamine
<u>Tryptophan</u>	Glycine*
Valine	Proline*
	Serine
	Tyrosine*
*Conditionally essential <u>Anti-metabolic</u>	

Table 3.2: List of the 20 natural amino acids, grouped into essential and non-essential amino acids. Conditionally essential amino acids can become essential during infancy, growth, and in states of disease. Three amino acids (tryptophan, methionine, and cysteine) inhibit the metabolic rate.

High-and Low-Quality Protein

The nutritional value of a protein-rich food is dependent on what amino acids it contains and in what quantities. A food that provides all of the essential amino acids in adequate amounts is called a complete protein source, while one that lacks one or more essential amino acids is called an incomplete protein source (Open Oregon Educational Science, 2020a)

Animal proteins are "complete," meaning they supply all the essential amino acids your body needs in the required amounts. Additionally, the body easily absorbs animal protein (Diet Doctor, 2024b).

In contrast, most plant proteins, with the exception of soy, are "incomplete" because they lack one or more essential amino acids. Therefore, vegans need to combine different plant-based proteins to ensure they get all the essential amino acids (Diet Doctor, 2024b).

Moreover, a significant problem with plant-based proteins is the presence of tannins and phytic acid. These compounds bind to proteins, and the high dietary fiber content in plants further reduces protein digestibility, resulting in low bioavailability of plant-based protein (Reid-McCann RJ, 2022).

Consequently, even if a food label lists a certain protein content, the actual amount of protein absorbed from some plant foods might be considerably lower. Practically, this means you might need to consume 20-50% more plant proteins to absorb the same amount of amino acids as from animal protein sources (Diet Doctor, 2024b).

As a result of these distinctions many researchers consider plant-based proteins to be of lower or variable quality, while animal-based proteins are deemed to be of higher quality (Reid-McCann RJ, 2022).

In addition, Dr. Ray Peat emphasized that many plant-based protein sources directly inhibit thyroid function and harm your hormonal balance—a subject I will discuss in detail in the next section.

Dr. Ray Peat did recommend a few plant-based protein sources, but generally, the proteins that are part of the Ray Peat diet framework come from an animal source, which provides your body with all the necessary amino acids. However, as will be discussed later in this chapter, muscle meat is especially high in antimetabolic amino acids, which is why a high-meat diet is not recommended for adults. In the remainder of this chapter, I will explore plant and animal-based protein sources through the lens of Dr. Ray Peat's nutritional research.

Benedicte Mai Lerche MSc PhD

Harmful Plant Proteins

Plant-based proteins especially soy products, lentils, beans, peas, nuts, almonds, and seeds such as quinoa, chia, and hemp seeds are being promoted as healthy and climate-friendly alternatives to animal-based protein (Medical News Today, 2023a).

However, Dr. Ray Peat emphasized that these plant-based proteins are harmful to your metabolic rate and hormonal balance.

Almonds, nuts, seeds, and grains contain high amounts of polyunsaturated fats (PUFAs) and amygdalin, both of which inhibit thyroid function (Peat R., Nutrition for Women: 100 Short Articles, 2001d, p. 17)

Beans, soybeans, green peas, chickpeas, lentils, and so forth are members of the legume family, which are rich in phytoestrogens (Medical News Today, 2023b; Peat R., Natural estrogens, 2008b).

Phytoestrogens are compounds produced by plants that exert estrogenic effects in humans (Medical News Today, 2018). Dr. Ray Peat noted that all legumes possess phytoestrogens, with all parts of

the plant containing some of these estrogenic compounds (Peat R., Natural estrogens, 2008b).
As mentioned, estrogen is a strong thyroid suppressor, as seen in Table 1.1 (Peat R., Progesterone in Orthomolecular Medicine, 2001c, p. 17; Peat R., From PMS to Menopause: Female Hormones in Context, 2001b, p. 78).

In addition, Dr. Ray Peat emphasized that beans, seeds, and grains contain indigestible fibers, that feed gut bacteria, leading to the overproduction of endotoxins and intestinal irritation (Functional Performance, 2012).

Key Points – Plant vs Animal Protein:

Protein consists of amino acids.

Animal protein sources generally contain a broader spectrum of amino acids than plant protein.

Animal protein is easily digested and has a high bioavailability compared to plant protein.

Common plant protein sources like nuts, seeds, and legumes contain amygdalin, PUFAs and phytoestrogens, which harm the metabolic rate.

Animal protein is generally considered of higher quality compared to plant protein.

A few plant protein sources are comparable to animal protein. These include potatoes and mushrooms.

Muscle meat has a high content of anti-metabolic amino acids, and excessive meat eating in adulthood is discouraged.

Benedicte Mai Lerche MSc PhD

Potatoes & Mushroom Protein

According to Dr. Ray Peat, only a few plant-based proteins match the quality of animal proteins, specifically, he mentioned well-cooked white potatoes and mushrooms (Ray Peat Clips, 2016x).

Potato protein:

Although widely recognized for their starch content, it's less well-known that potatoes are an excellent source of high-quality protein.

Potatoes are rich in both amino acids and keto-acids, which are found in the fluid surrounding the starch grains (Peat R., Nutrition for Women: 100 Short Articles, 2001d, p. 99). The body can convert keto-acids into essential amino acids, making potatoes an excellent source of protein (Peat R., Tryptophan, serotonin, and aging, 2006d; Expulsia, 2011).

Potato protein is highly digestible and has a balanced amino acid composition. The protein quality of potatoes is comparable to that of eggs and milk (Food Research International, 2021).

On a weight basis, potatoes and milk provide comparable protein levels. Specifically, one kilogram (around two pounds) of potatoes delivers approximately 33 grams of protein, an amount similar to what is found in one liter (a quarter gallon) of milk *(50k-food health, 2011)*.

Dr. Peat recommended white potatoes, not sweet potatoes, as sweet potatoes have a high carotene content, which, as mentioned, suppresses thyroid function, see Table 1.1 (Ray Peat Clips, 2014a).

According to Peat, the optimal way to consume white potatoes is to boil them thoroughly and eat them with generous amounts of salt and saturated fats like butter or coconut oil. This helps prevent the starch from causing blood sugar disturbances and digestive irritation (Peat R., Ray Peat Eluv Radio 2014 Stress and Trauma, 2017).

The keto-acids in potatoes can be used as fuel by the brain and heart cells, instead of sugar (George F Cahill Jr, 2003). In the case of an emergency stress situation, keto-acids can be very helpful, as they provide energy and essential amino acids without stimulating insulin secretion (Another School of Thought Radio, 2011).

Dr. Ray Peat recommended using potato juice in cases of severe stress or digestive issues. Juicing raw peeled potatoes (using an electric juicer) removes the starch grains and creates a juice that is very rich in keto-acids, with a protein value comparable to that of egg yolk (Another School of Thought Radio, 2011; Peat R., From PMS to Menopause: Female Hormones in Context, 2001b, p. 129).

The juice can be cooked in coconut oil or butter to make something like scrambled eggs. The juice can also be made into a soup with the addition of water, salt, onions, and spices. However, it's important to avoid boiling the soup to prevent it from coagulating (Ray Peat clips, 2014b).

Mushroom protein:

Mushrooms are a unique vegetable that offers high amounts of premium protein (Peat R., Mushrooms-observations and interpretations, 2015). Dr. Ray Peat highlighted that the protein found in mushrooms is easily assimilated and has a quality similar to animal protein sources (Ray Peat Clips, 2016x).

Besides their high-quality protein, mushrooms also contain beneficial nutrients and compounds with anti-estrogenic, anti-inflammatory, and antimicrobial properties (Peat R., Mushrooms-observations and interpretations, 2015).

Due to their antimicrobial effect, Dr. Peat explained that mushrooms can be used instead of raw carrots or bamboo shoots to cleanse the intestines (Roddy, 2016).

Because of their numerous benefits, Dr. Peat frequently consumed mushrooms (Roddy, 2016).

However, it's crucial to mention that mushrooms contain compounds that are toxic to the liver. These toxins are neutralized by heat, leading Dr. Ray Peat to advise boiling your mushrooms for 1-3 hours (Peat R., Mushrooms-observations and interpretations, 2015).

Once boiled, the mushrooms can be utilized in preparing soups, or they can be fried in coconut oil to achieve a crispy texture. While numerous varieties of mushrooms exist, Dr. Peat typically recommended white button mushrooms as a safe option (Peat R., Mushrooms-observations and interpretations, 2015).

Key Points – Potatoes & Mushrooms:

White potatoes and white button mushrooms are safe and healthy vegetable protein sources.

White potatoes should be thoroughly cooked (boiled) and eaten with saturated fats and salt.

Juicing the potatoes and cooking the juice create a meal high in keto acids, which have anti-stress effects.

White button mushrooms should be cooked (boiled) thoroughly (1-3 hours) to destroy their liver toxins.

White button mushrooms have anti-microbial properties and can be used in lieu of raw carrot and cooked bamboo shoots.

Benedicte Mai Lerche MSc PhD

Why Eggs are Superfoods

Dr. Ray Peat explained that eggs are an excellent source of high-quality protein (Thyroid Patient Advocacy, 2024). It's crucial to avoid overcooking eggs because the small amount of polyunsaturated fats (PUFAs) they contain can become oxidized with excessive heat. Therefore, soft-boiled eggs are preferable to hard-boiled eggs, etc. (Ray Peat Clips, 2023).

A large egg offers approximately 6 grams of protein, along with essential vitamins and minerals such as Vitamin A, B vitamins, Choline, Selenium, and Zinc, as well as Vitamins D and E (HealthLine, 2022)

Select the best eggs:

The flavor of eggs can significantly change based on the chickens' diet. For example, a noticeable fishy taste in eggs indicates that the chickens were fed a diet high in polyunsaturated fats, which results in eggs with a higher concentration of PUFAs (Get Cracking, 2023). In such cases, selecting a different brand of eggs is important.

Sometimes, these eggs with high PUFA content are marketed as healthier options and sold under the label of "Omega-3-Enhanced" Eggs, which contain up to twelve times more PUFAs than regular eggs *(Lam, 2022)*.

Dr. Ray Peat explained that it is important to select cage-free eggs, as chickens confined in cages experience stress, which can negatively impact the nutritional quality of their eggs (Ray Peat Clips, 2010b).

Pastured eggs which are sometimes referred to as "grass-fed," are likely superior to other egg varieties. Pastured eggs are laid by chickens that are raised on the green pasture, with access to sun, bugs, space, and fresh air. The chickens eat a natural diet of grass, bugs, and greens (Lam, 2022).

Key Points – Eggs:

Eggs are a great source of high-quality protein.

Don't overcook your eggs.

Select cage-free eggs.

Avoid eggs that have a fishy taste (they are high in PUFAs).

Types and Amounts of Meat & Fish

Ruminant meats and white fish are low in PUFAs and provide high-quality protein, delivering about 20 grams of protein per 100 grams (approximately 3.5 ounces), as detailed in Table 3.1 (Health Line, 2023; Britannica, 2024).

Avoid oily fish:

Oily fish, such as herring, mackerel, salmon, and tuna, are rich in PUFAs (omega-3 fatty acids) and should be avoided. Instead, opt for white fish like cod, haddock, pollock, flounder, and halibut (Peat R., The Great Fish Oil Experiment, 2007c).

Choose meats of ruminants:

Non-ruminant animals, such as pigs and poultry, store PUFAs from their feed in their tissues, making it essential to avoid or limit their consumption unless you are certain they haven't been fed a diet high in PUFAs (Ray Peat Clips, 2016g).

Contrary to popular belief, pork fat (lard) is not highly saturated. In the USA and other industrialized countries, pigs are often fed on corn and soybeans, which contain enough polyunsaturated fatty acids (PUFAs) to make lard as unsaturated as harmful seed oils (Peat R., From PMS to Menopause: Female Hormones in Context, 2001b, p. 154).

Ruminant animals, such as cattle, bison, sheep, goats, and deer, do not accumulate fats from their feed in their fat tissue. As a result, the fat of ruminant animals (tallow) is highly saturated. This is why Dr. Ray Peat recommended the consumption of ruminant meats over pork, chicken, turkey, and other non-ruminant meats (Ray Peat Clips, 2016g).

Vitamins and minerals in meat and fish:

Ruminant meats and white fish are excellent sources of B vitamins, vitamin A, vitamin D, magnesium, potassium, zinc, selenium, etc. (Britannica, 2024). Calf and beef liver, however, are even stronger sources of essential vitamins and minerals, a subject I will return to later in this chapter.

Thyroid-suppressing amino acids:

Dr. Broda Barnes detailed how consuming excessive amounts of protein could inhibit thyroid function (Barnes & Galton, 1976, pp. 273-274). Dr. Ray Peat clarified that it is the amino acids cysteine, methionine, and tryptophan that have this dampening effect on metabolism (Peat R.,

Tryptophan, serotonin, and aging, 2006d; Peat R., Gelatin, stress, longevity, 2004). These amino acids are found in abundance in muscle meat, meaning the finer cuts of meat and fish (Ray Peat Clips, 2010a; Thyroid Patient Advocacy, 2024).

Additionally, Dr. Ray Peat highlighted that methionine and tryptophan contribute to aging. Research indicates that reducing the intake of these amino acids can promote longevity (Ray Peat Clips, 2010a).

The dietary needs for cysteine, methionine, and tryptophan decrease significantly in adulthood (Peat R., Gelatin, stress, longevity, 2004). However, most adults who consume meat and fish ingest excessively high quantities of these three amino acids (Peat R., Nutrition for Women: 100 Short Articles, 2001d, p. 81; Ray Peat Clips, 2010a).

Dr. Ray Peat recommended that the muscle meat of ruminants and white fish should be moderated in adulthood to about 1-2 ounces (30-60 grams) daily (Ray Peat Clips, 2010a). Personally, I eat muscle meat only a couple of times per week on average.

Historically, we consumed the whole animal, ingesting a significant amount of gelatin alongside muscle meat. As I will detail in the following section, gelatin offers a more thyroid-friendly amino acid profile. By replacing some of your muscle meat with gelatin-rich meats and gelatin powders, you can limit the intake of the three anti-thyroid and age-promoting amino acids (Peat R., Gelatin, stress, longevity, 2004).

The Benefits of Gelatin

Gelatin, the cooked form of collagen, is sourced from a range of animal parts including skin, tendons, ears, snouts, tails, and the tough bony cuts of meat (Peat R., Gelatin, stress, longevity, 2004).

Unlike muscle meat, gelatin provides an amino acid profile beneficial for thyroid health and longevity, as it lacks tryptophan and contains only minimal cysteine and methionine. Instead, gelatin is abundant in glycine, known for its anti-inflammatory properties (Peat R., Gelatin, stress, longevity, 2004).

Dr. Ray Peat recommended limiting the finer cuts of meat and fish (muscle meat) and instead consuming foods like gelatin powder, bone broth, oxtail soup, and tough and bony cuts of ruminant meats (Peat R., Gelatin, stress, longevity, 2004; Ray Peat Clips, 2010a; Peat R., Tryptophan, serotonin, and aging, 2006d).

He also recommended consuming 10-20 grams of gelatin powder alongside a meal rich in muscle meat, such as steak or fish. This approach helps ensure a balanced absorption of amino acids into the bloodstream (Peat R., Gelatin, stress, longevity,

2004; Peat R., Tryptophan, serotonin, and aging, 2006d).

Oxtail soup and bone broth are both rich sources of gelatin. For the bone broth, it is important to use bones with attached cartilage, ligaments, and tendons, near joints and avoid the long marrow bones, because of the high iron content in the marrow (Expulsia, 2024a).

Dr. Ray Peat emphasizes that iron is a potentially toxic metal that we often ingest in excess. Consuming excessive amounts of iron can result in various health problems (Peat R., 2006f). To release the gelatin from the bones, it is advised to cook your bone broth for about 3 hours.

Asian grocery stores often carry traditional foods rich in gelatin, including prepared pig skin, ears, tails, and chicken feet. You can also find gelatin in marshmallows and gummy bears—but make sure to check the label (Peat R., Gelatin, stress, longevity, 2004).

Pure gelatin, available in powder or sheets from pork or beef without additives, offers a convenient way to incorporate gelatin into your diet. As a fat-free product, pork gelatin contains no PUFAs.

It's important to fully dissolve gelatin before consumption, which can be done by mixing it with boiling water or milk. You can also melt it in the microwave instead. Once dissolved, gelatin can be added to a wide range of foods, including custards, mousses, ice cream, soups, sauces, cheesecakes, pies, and more. It can also be mixed with fruit juices for desserts or juice concentrate to make gummy bear-like candies (Peat R., Gelatin, stress, longevity, 2004).

Gelatin has gelling properties when it cools down. In contrast, hydrolyzed gelatin can be dissolved directly in cold drinks such as orange juice and it has no gelling properties (OnePeak Medical, 2024)..

Hydrolyzed gelatin powder is also called collagen hydrolysate or collagen peptides. It is a form of gelatin that has undergone more processing to break down the proteins into smaller fragments (OnePeak Medical, 2024).

Using hydrolyzed gelatin should be fine and convenient, but I prefer regular gelatin. When Dr. Ray Peat discussed the benefits of gelatin, he always referred to regular gelatin. He was not a fan of hydrolyzed proteins in general, advocating for foods as close to their natural state as possible.

I prefer Great Lakes Gelatin as my go-to brand for gelatin powder. However, supermarkets often carry gelatin powders or sheets, which are fine too.

How much gelatin powder is safe:

As mentioned earlier in this chapter, both men and women require approximately 100 grams of protein daily. Dr. Ray Peat emphasized that for adults, a significant portion of this protein requirement can be met by incorporating gelatin powder into the diet. This approach helps fulfill protein needs without an excess of thyroid-suppressing amino acids (tryptophan, cysteine, and methionine) (Peat R., Gelatin, stress, longevity, 2004).

Gelatin powder contains about 86 grams of protein per 100 grams (US Department of Agriculture, 2018). I aim to include 1-2 tablespoons of gelatin in my daily diet, which provides roughly 11-22 grams of protein. However, larger daily amounts of gelatin can also be safely consumed (Great Lakes Wellness, 2014).

However, it's important to note that the amino acid profile of gelatin is not optimal for growing children, and excessive consumption of gelatin may not be ideal for kids, as it could replace other essential foods (Peat R., Gelatin, stress, longevity, 2004).

> ### Key Points – Meat, Fish & Gelatin:
>
> Avoid or limit meat from non-ruminant animals like pork and poultry.
>
> Avoid oily fish like salmon, tuna, mackerel, etc.
>
> Eat meat from ruminant animals such as beef and lamb.
>
> Eat white fish like cod, haddock, flounder, etc.
>
> Muscle meat (the fine cuts of meat) is rich in the amino acids: cysteine, methionine, and tryptophan which suppress thyroid function and promote aging.
>
> Adults should limit their muscle meat intake and instead focus on gelatinous cuts of meat, bone broth, oxtail soup, gelatin powder, etc.

Benedicte Mai Lerche MSc PhD

Become a Happy Milk Drinker

Dr. Ray Peat highly endorses the consumption of milk, cheese, and non-sour yogurt, emphasizing these dairy products as sources of high-quality protein and calcium (Peat R., Milk in context: allergies, ecology, and some myths, 2011). He generally recommended consuming grass-fed, organic milk and typically preferred low-fat (1% or 2%) skimmed varieties (Herb Doctors, 2018).

How much milk daily:

Peat was a dedicated consumer of milk, often drinking up to half a gallon (almost two liters) daily. However, acknowledging that such a quantity might not be suitable for everyone, Dr. Peat typically recommended a daily intake of a quart of a gallon (nearly 1 liter) of skimmed milk, providing approximately 32 grams of protein (Thyroid Patient Advocacy, 2024).

The benefits of low-fat dairy products:

As the fat content in milk, yogurt, and cheese increases, the protein concentration per 100 grams slightly decreases. By choosing skimmed milk and opting for low-fat versions of cheese and yogurt, you can increase your daily protein and calcium intake without exceeding your calorie budget. Additionally, low-fat dairy products are valuable for weight loss efforts. More information on this topic will be discussed in the following section.

Hormones in milk:

A common concern among individuals is the presence of hormones in milk. There is a minimal quantity of estrogen in milk (Herb Doctors, 2018). However, Dr. Ray Peat pointed out that milk boasts a progesterone content that is twentyfold higher than its estrogen levels (Thyroid Patient Advocacy, 2024; Herb Doctors, 2018). Moreover, milk even includes a slight amount of thyroid hormone. Overall, milk is deemed highly advantageous for improving the metabolic rate in both men and women (Thyroid Patient Advocacy, 2024).

Pasteurized and homogenized milk vs raw milk:

Some individuals regard pasteurized and homogenized milk as problematic, favoring raw milk instead. Dr. Ray Peat highlighted the high nutritional value of raw milk. However, he also clarified that homogenization should not be a significant concern, as our digestive systems undertake a comparable process (Herb Doctors, 2018). He further stressed that pasteurization, a quick heating process, is vital for eliminating any bacteria in the milk (Herb Doctors, 2018).

Allergies and milk:

Numerous people report allergic reactions to milk, which could be due to several factors.

In the United States, reduced-fat milk must be fortified with vitamins A and D, introducing potential allergens through the additives used in vitamin formulations. Therefore, whole milk tends to have a lower likelihood of causing allergic reactions (Peat R., Milk in context: allergies, ecology, and some myths, 2011).

Moreover, carrageenan, a widely used thickener in dairy products, is identified by Dr. Ray Peat as a significant allergen and a very harmful substance (Peat R., Milk in context: allergies, ecology, and some myths, 2011).

Lactose intolerance:

Another common issue is lactose intolerance. People who are lactose intolerant cannot break down lactose (milk sugar). As a result, lactose proceeds undigested to the large intestine, where it attracts water and undergoes fermentation by bacteria. This process can lead to symptoms like bloating and diarrhea (Open Oregon, 2020c).

In lactose intolerance, there is a deficiency in the digestive enzyme called lactase, which is needed to break down the disaccharide lactose into its monosaccharides, glucose, and galactose. (Open Oregon, 2020c).

To mitigate lactose intolerance, Dr. Ray Peat recommended a gradual reintroduction of milk into the diet (Peat R., Milk in context: allergies, ecology, and some myths, 2011). He advises beginning with half a cup of milk at each main meal, a method that can promote lactase enzyme production over two to three weeks (Peat R., Milk in context: allergies, ecology, and some myths, 2011).

It's crucial to note that lactose intolerance can also stem from bacterial overgrowth, hypothyroidism, and progesterone deficiency (Peat R., Milk in context: allergies, ecology, and some myths, 2011; Herb Doctors, 2018).

In my experience, eliminating lactose intolerance completely can be very challenging, and Dr. Ray Peat did not oppose drinking lactose-free milk. In lactose-free milk, the lactase enzyme is added to the milk, thereby predigesting the lactose (Herb Doctors, 2018).

Different types of milk:

People with different forms of milk allergies may find Ultra-High Temperature (UHT) milk a more tolerable alternative. UHT milk is heated to a higher temperature than traditionally pasteurized milk, potentially slightly reducing its vitamin and mineral content and changing its flavor. However, some people report that UHT milk is easier to digest (Expulsia, 2011)

Dr. Peat observed that individuals with milk-related digestive issues sometimes find relief by switching milk brands (Peat R., Milk in context: allergies, ecology, and some myths, 2011). Alternatively, choosing goat's milk over cow's milk is another option. Some people who have adverse reactions to cow's milk discover they can better tolerate goat's milk (Herb Doctors, 2018).

Non-sour yogurt:

Dr. Ray Peat had a preference for Greek yogurt over regular yogurt because of its lower lactic acid content. He highlighted the importance of avoiding or minimizing the consumption of sour yogurts, kefir, and other products rich in lactic acid (Herb Doctors, 2018).

Lactic acid promotes inflammation and depletes the liver's glycogen stores, thereby lowering blood sugar (Ray Peat Clips, 2016i). Dr. Peat explained that excessive intake of lactic acid-rich products may result in fatigue, headaches, migraines, and other symptoms, especially in those with compromised thyroid function (Ray Peat Clips, 2016k).

If you can find a Greek yogurt that isn't overly sour, it means it has had much of its lactic acid strained out. The straining process also eliminates the majority of the lactose, making Greek yogurt suitable for people with lactose intolerance. In the USA, there's a brand of Greek yogurt called "FAGE yogurt" that comes recommended.

The Importance of Calcium

Parathyroid hormone (PTH), released by the parathyroid glands, regulates calcium levels in the blood. Dr. Ray Peat emphasized that elevated PTH also inhibits metabolism and promotes aging and inflammation (Peat R., Calcium and Disease: Hypertension, organ calcification, & shock, vs. respiratory energy, 2009b).

When your calcium intake is insufficient, PTH levels rise, drawing calcium from your bones into your bloodstream, which can lead to osteoporosis and calcification of soft tissues. Conversely, a high dietary intake of calcium suppresses PTH secretion, preventing the release of calcium from the bones (Cleveland Clinic, 2021; Peat R., Calcium and Disease: Hypertension, organ calcification, & shock, vs. respiratory energy, 2009b).

Additionally, it is important to mention that phosphate promotes the secretion of PTH. Dr. Ray Peat emphasized the importance of a diet high in calcium and low in phosphate (Ray Peat, 2013).

Foods naturally highest in phosphate relative to calcium include cereals, legumes, nuts, seeds, meats, and fish. Many prepared foods also contain added phosphate.

Foods with a higher, safer ratio of calcium to phosphate are dairy, masa harina tortillas, fruits, and well-cooked green leafy vegetables (Ray Peat, 2013).

The benefits of a diet rich in calcium:

To suppress the release of PTH you need about 2000 mg of calcium daily. Supplementing vitamin D and K will also help suppress the PTH level (KMUD, 2012; Peat R., Calcium and Disease: Hypertension, organ calcification, & shock, vs. respiratory energy, 2009b).

By suppressing the secretion of PTH, a diet rich in calcium promotes your metabolic rate, helps prevent aging, and inflammation, and safeguards against osteoporosis. In addition, dietary calcium also plays a direct role in combating obesity as calcium inhibits the fat-synthesizing enzyme, fatty acid synthase (Peat R., Calcium and Disease: Hypertension, organ calcification, & shock, vs. respiratory energy, 2009b; Functional Performance Systems, 2011b).

Calcium content in dairy:

Milk, cheese, and Greek yogurt are excellent sources of both protein and calcium. Dr. Ray Peat recommended obtaining much of the daily protein from dairy products and limiting meat intake (KMUD, 2012).

Meat and fish are high in phosphate, which promotes PTH secretion. In addition, muscle meats are rich in thyroid-suppressing amino acids (KMUD, 2012).

In other words, dairy products enhance your metabolic rate and support healthy weight loss more effectively than meat and fish. Thus, focusing on dairy as your main source of protein is a cornerstone of the "Ray Peat diet" (KMUD, 2012).

Eggshell calcium:

For those less inclined to consume large amounts of dairy, eggshell powder offers an excellent calcium source. Dr. Ray Peat endorsed eggshells as the best type of calcium supplement (Ray Peat Clips KMUD, 2016c).

In many store-bought calcium supplements, calcium is bound to a counterion that may contribute to bone demineralization. In contrast, eggshells contain calcium in the form of calcium carbonate, the primary mineral in newly formed bone (Ray Peat Clips KMUD, 2016c).

To make your own calcium supplement, you can use either white or brown eggshells that have been rinsed and boiled to eliminate any bacteria. After boiling, the eggshells should be dried in the oven at low heat to avoid burning. Once dry, they can be ground into a fine powder using a coffee grinder (Ray Peat Clips KMUD, 2016c).

Consuming 3/4 teaspoon of powdered eggshells daily will meet Dr. Ray Peat's recommended calcium intake of approximately 2000 mg. It is best to take ¼ teaspoon with each main meal (Ray Peat Clips KMUD, 2016c).

For many people, it is beneficial to use both dairy products and eggshell powder to achieve a daily calcium intake of about 2000 mg.

Other foods rich in calcium:

As mentioned in the last chapter, Dr. Ray Peat was very fond of corn tortillas made from lime-treated corn (masa harina flour). Besides being a safe starch and an excellent substitute for bread, these tortillas are also rich in calcium. The lime, or calcium hydroxide, used in treating the corn enriches it with calcium, making tortillas made from masa harina flour a valuable calcium source (Jorge L. Rosado, 2005).

The longer the corn is treated with lime, the higher the calcium content of the flour. Commercially bought masa harina often doesn't compare to the traditional 12 hours of lime treatment, but it still contains about 30 mg of calcium per 30 g of flour (Jorge L. Rosado, 2005).

Well-cooked leafy green vegetables, such as kale, turnip greens, beet greens and collared (spring) greens, are excellent sources of calcium. Many fruits also contain calcium; for example, figs are a rich source (BHOF, 2024; International Osteoporosis Foundation, 2024).

Table 3.3 provides the calcium content of some foods, which are part of the "Ray Peat diet" guidelines.

Food	Serving size	Serving size	Calcium Content
Milk	¼ gallon	1 liter	1200 mg
Greek yogurt	6 oz	170 g	220 mg
Hard cheeses*	1 oz	28 g	240 mg
Mozzarella	4 oz	113 g	450mg
Feta cheese	4 oz	113 g	540 mg
Masa Harina flour	1/3 cup	30 g	30 mg
Figs, dried	2 figs		65 mg
Eggshell powder	¾ teaspoon		2000 mg
Cooked leafy greens	100 g		80-250 mg

Table 3.3: The calcium content of some pro-metabolic foods. *Hard cheeses e.g. Cheddar, Parmesan, Emmental, and Gruyere. (International Osteoporosis Foundation, 2024; BHOF, 2024; Ray Peat Clips KMUD, 2016c).

Key Points – The Importance of Calcium:

Elevated parathyroid hormone (PTH) levels can cause osteoporosis, premature aging, inflammation, and slow metabolism.

Diets low in calcium and high in phosphate increase PTH levels.

Consuming 2000 mg of calcium daily helps maintain low PTH levels.

Dairy products, including milk, cheese, and Greek yogurt, are excellent sources of both protein and calcium.

Dairy is a more pro-metabolic protein source compared to meat and fish, which are high in phosphate.

Other calcium-rich foods include masa harina tortillas, cooked green leafy vegetables, and fruits like figs.

Powdered eggshells can serve as an effective calcium supplement.

Shellfish and Liver as Superfoods

Dr. Ray Peat advised having a serving of 2-3 ounces (approximately 56-85 grams.) of shellfish and about 4 ounces (approximately 113 grams) of beef or calf liver once a week (KMUD: Food, 2016; Eluv Radio 2014 Stress and Trauma, 2014b; #55: Bioenergetic Nutrition Basics I, 2021).

Shellfish:

Shellfish such as shrimp, oysters, clams, mussels, scallops, and lobster offer high-quality protein and essential trace minerals that support thyroid function including, selenium, iodine, and copper (Wilson, 2015, p. 26; Peat R., From PMS to Menopause: Female Hormones in Context, 2001b, pp. 171-172).

It is crucial to consume shellfish that have lived in the sea, as farmed shellfish lack beneficial trace minerals. Additionally, it is important to avoid shellfish and fish with added colorants and preservatives.

According to Dr. Ray Peat, avoiding iodine supplements and even iodized salt is important, as these often provide excessive amounts of iodine. Dr.

Peat warned that large, continuous doses of iodine, around 0.5-1 mg daily, can cause inflammation and even cancer in the thyroid gland. The best way to obtain the right amount of iodine is by consuming shellfish once or more per week (Ryan Heeney, 2019)

Beef or calf liver:

In many cultures, organ meats, including kidneys, heart, tongue, and liver, are considered delicacies, with the liver being particularly rich in nutrients. Beef liver is often called the superfood of the animal kingdom because it is one of the most nutrient-dense foods on earth. It provides about 26 grams of protein per 100 grams and ample amounts of important nutrients, including B vitamins and other pro-metabolic nutrients like vitamins A, D, E, and K, as well as copper, zinc, selenium, and manganese (Web MD, 2023; Very Well Fit, 2022; Enviromedica, 2024; Britannica, 2024).

If you do not enjoy liver, taking a B-complex supplement can be beneficial, as B vitamins are especially important for liver function. The liver is the main organ responsible for converting the inactive thyroid hormone T4 into the active T3 (see Table 1.1).

Key Points – Shellfish & Liver as Superfoods

Shellfish are rich in trace minerals, which are important for good thyroid function.

It is advised to have a serving of 2-3 ounces (56-85 grams) of shellfish once or more per week.

Beef and calf liver are great sources of important vitamins such as B vitamins, which are essential for liver function and thereby thyroid function.

It is advised to eat about 4 ounces (113 grams) of beef or calf liver once a week.

If you do not enjoy liver, taking a B-complex supplement daily can be beneficial.

Benedicte Mai Lerche MSc PhD

Veganism & The Ray Peat Diet

Many wonder if following the "Ray Peat diet" is practical for vegans. Veganism involves consuming exclusively plant-based foods, excluding all animal-derived products. Previously in this chapter, I have outlined some of the issues with plant proteins, which are summarized below.

Vegan diets often include plant proteins such as almonds, nuts, seeds, and grains, which contain high amounts of PUFAs and amygdalin, both of which inhibit thyroid function (Peat R., Nutrition for Women: 100 Short Articles, 2001d, p. 17)

Additionally, vegan diets commonly incorporate legumes like beans, soybeans, soy products, green peas, chickpeas, and lentils, which are rich in phytoestrogens (Medical News Today, 2023b; Peat R., Natural estrogens, 2008b).

Furthermore, plant-based proteins are generally harder to digest and less bioavailable compared to animal-based sources. Consequently, even if a food label lists a certain protein content, the actual amount of protein absorbed from some plant foods might be considerably lower, necessitating larger quantities of food to meet the daily protein requirement of approximately 100 grams (Diet Doctor, 2024b).

Therefore, the typical vegan diet may adversely affect metabolic rate and overall hormonal balance.

It is indeed possible to follow the "Ray Peat diet" as a vegan if you rely on potatoes and mushrooms for protein. However, you'll need to consume them in significant amounts (Ray Peat Clips, 2016x).
For example, to satisfy your protein requirements with just potatoes, you'd need about five pounds daily (Ray Peat Clips, 2016j). Juicing the potatoes might be a practical approach to concentrate their protein.

Vegans often become deficient in calcium since they do not consume dairy (Ray Peat Clips, 2016x). To ensure adequate calcium intake, vegans could incorporate well-cooked leafy green vegetables. As discussed in Chapter 3, these vegetables contain anti-nutrients. By thoroughly cooking leafy green vegetables, it is possible to take advantage of their calcium content while limiting the effects of their anti-nutrients (Eluv Radio: Stress and Trauma, 2014a).

Adopting Dr. Peat's diet principles as a vegan is doable, though it comes with certain challenges.

For vegetarians, it is easier due to the inclusion of proteins from dairy, and possibly eggs and shellfish.

Emphasizing substantial amounts of milk and other dairy products in your diet provides the added benefit of high calcium intake, which is crucial for keeping the parathyroid hormone down into a safe range, which is important for optimal metabolism and longevity.

Incorporate dairy, potatoes, mushrooms, eggs, and shellfish taps into a wealth of superfoods that support the metabolic rate. A vegetarian approach also offers the advantage of lower levels of age-promoting and thyroid-suppressing amino acids and phosphate, which are found in abundance in muscle meat and the meat of fish.

The key takeaway is that meat consumption isn't essential for adults. I follow a vegetarian variant of Dr. Peat's diet most days, focusing on proteins from dairy, eggs, shrimp, potatoes, and mushrooms. However, I do include meat or fish in my diet once or twice per week on average and also integrate gelatine.

Benedicte Mai Lerche MSc PhD

Protein & Blood Sugar

It's a common belief that only carbohydrates affect blood sugar, but it's crucial to understand that consuming a large amount of protein on its own can also dramatically disrupt blood sugar (Another School of Thought Radio, 2011).

When we eat protein, it is broken down by digestive enzymes into its amino acids, some of these amino acids strongly stimulate insulin secretion. Insulin helps cells absorb these amino acids to create new proteins. However, insulin also lowers blood sugar, so consuming protein without balancing it with healthy carbohydrates can cause a sharp drop in blood sugar (Another School of Thought Radio, 2011; Functional Performance Systems, 2024a).

This means that eating pure protein alone, like consuming pure starch (glucose), overstimulates insulin and subsequently lowers blood sugar.

Throughout this book, I have explained that low blood sugar is detrimental to your metabolic rate. It directly impairs the liver's ability to turn T4 into T3 and sets in motion a stress response involving the secretion of adrenalin and cortisol, that further dampens metabolism.

Protein from meat, fish, eggs, gelatine, etc. should always be accompanied by an abundant amount of healthy carbohydrates. Refer to Chapter 3 for a list of good carbohydrates (Another School of Thought Radio, 2011).

Orange juice is one of Dr. Ray Peat's favorite carbohydrates and is a great option to accompany your proteins. However, the high vitamin C content in oranges promotes iron absorption from food. Since iron is a potentially toxic metal that we usually consume in excess, Dr. Ray Peat recommended avoiding drinking orange juice with red meat and liver, which are especially rich in iron (Peat R., 2006f).

Dr. Ray Peat also suggested consuming fruits before a large protein meal to ensure the liver is stocked with glycogen, preventing blood sugar from falling when consuming a large amount of protein (Ray Peat Clips, 2016o). For example, you could have some grape or berry juice about 20 minutes before a high-protein meal.

It's important to note that milk is a complete meal in itself, containing protein, fat, and milk sugar. Therefore, dairy doesn't disturb blood sugar and doesn't need to be balanced with other foods.

High-protein, low-carbohydrate diets:

Many people who see sugar, honey, sweet fruits, etc as unhealthy and who advocate for high-protein, low-carbohydrate diets such as paleo, carnivore, and ketogenic types diets do not understand that eating large amounts of protein without enough carbohydrates can hurt their metabolic rate and lead to chronically elevated cortisol.

If the diet is very high in protein and very low in carbohydrates, cortisol tends to become chronically elevated. As explained in Chapter 3, cortisol converts protein from the diet and muscles into glucose. Since glucose is essential for brain, nerve, and organ function, the body will need to produce glucose if the diet lacks it (Another School of Thought Radio, 2011). Paradoxically, chronically high cortisol can lead to a state where protein is excessively converted into glucose, resulting in chronically elevated blood glucose—a situation that can be mistaken for diabetes. Cortisol is a catabolic hormone, meaning it breaks down tissues, and chronically elevated cortisol will therefore contribute to muscle loss, tissue wasting, and premature aging (Another School of Thought Radio, 2011; Ray Peat clips, 2016t).

List of Bad Protein

Avoid nuts, seeds, and grains:

- Almonds
- All nuts except for macadamia nuts.
- Chia, hemp, and all other seeds
- Quinoa and all other grains.

* Macadamia nuts are low in PUFA compared to most other nuts and can be eaten occasionally.

Avoid the legume family

- Beans
- Soybeans
- Tofu and all other soy products
- Green peas
- Chickpeas
- Lentils
- Peanuts
- And all other members of the legume family

Avoid oily fish:

- Herring
- Mackerel
- Salmon
- Tuna

Avoid or limit meat of non-ruminant animals:

- Pork
- Poultry

List of Good Proteins

Protein-rich vegetables:

- White potatoes (well-boiled)
- Potato juice (cooked)
- White button mushrooms (boiled for 1-3 hours)

Eggs:

- You can eat as many eggs as you want.
- Do not overcook your eggs
- Avoid eggs that taste like fish and
- Avoid eggs from caged chickens.
- Grounded eggshells make a great calcium supplement.

Dairy products from cows or goats:

- Cow's Milk (skimmed or whole)
- Goat's Milk
- Greek yogurt (2% or 10%)
- All cheeses without additives
- Ice cream made from natural ingredients (homemade or Häagen-Dazs)

Shellfish:

- Shrimp
- Oysters
- Crab
- Lobster
- Clams etc.

Shellfish are rich in thyroid-supporting trace minerals and should be eaten at least once a week. The shellfish must be wild-caught from the sea rather than farmed.

White fish:

- Cod
- Haddock
- Pollock
- Flounder
- Halibut etc.

Fish meat is classified as muscle meat, which should be limited to a maximum of 1-2 ounces (30-60 grams) daily on average.

Meat from ruminant animals:

- Beef
- Veal
- Goat
- Sheep
- Lamb
- Deer
- Beef or calf liver.

The fine cuts of ruminant meat are classified as muscle meat, which should be limited to a maximum of 1-2 ounces (30-60 grams) daily on average.

Gelatine:

- Bone broth, oxtail soup, etc.
- Gelatin powder from pork or beef

Benedicte Mai Lerche MSc PhD

Chapter 5: Salt & Spices

Benedicte Mai Lerche MSc PhD

Are You Getting Enough Salt?

We are frequently cautioned to restrict our salt intake due to concerns that it may lead to high blood pressure and water retention (edema). However, Dr. Ray Peat argued that the opposite is true; consuming insufficient salt can increase blood pressure and cause edema (Peat R., Salt, energy, metabolic rate, and longevity, 2016b; KMUD, 2011).

Dr. Ray Peat's perspective on salt was significantly shaped by the research conducted by Dr. Tom Brewer (Brewer, 2024)

Salt which is chemically known as sodium chloride, exerts an osmotic pressure that draws water from the tissues into the bloodstream. This role of salt is vital in sustaining blood volume, which is crucial for the effective transport of oxygen and nutrients to the cells. (Peat R., Salt, energy, metabolic rate, and longevity, 2016b; Brewer, 2024).

Consider this: Salt attracts water. Consuming too little salt lowers its concentration in the bloodstream, reducing the blood's ability to retain water. This causes water to seep out of the blood vessels into the tissues, leading to edema and reduced blood volume (Brewer, 2024).

The decreased blood volume lowers the delivery of oxygen and nutrients to tissues. Consequently, the body raises blood pressure to ensure adequate blood flow to the cells (Peat R., Salt, energy, metabolic rate, and longevity, 2016b; Peat R., Nutrition for Women: 100 Short Articles, 2001d, pp. I-II; Brewer, 2024).

Individuals with a slow metabolic rate often do not retain salt (sodium) effectively and frequently suffer from water-logged tissues (edema). Dr. Ray Peat noted that for those with hypothyroidism or suffering from PMS, increasing salt intake can be especially beneficial in preventing edema (KMUD: Blood Pressure Regulation Heart Failure and Muscle Atrophy , 2012; Peat R., Water: swelling, tension, pain, fatigue, aging, 2009d).

A diet with adequate salt supports metabolism, increases body temperature, protects against stress and inflammation, lowers adrenaline, improves sleep, and stabilizes blood sugar level (Peat R., Salt, energy, metabolic rate, and longevity, 2016b; KMUD, 2012).

Dr. Peat suggested using salt according to one's cravings and simply salting food to taste, essentially adding a little extra salt to various foods throughout the day (KMUD, 2011).

It's important to note that increasing your salt intake suddenly might require an adjustment period. Initially, you might retain more water for a few days. However, in the long term, a diet higher in salt will help prevent water retention (Peat R., Nutrition for Women: 100 Short Articles, 2001d, pp. I-II).

Benedicte Mai Lerche MSc PhD

Salt & Species

It's crucial to steer clear of Himalayan and Celtic salts, which are red and gray respectively, due to their content of iron and other potentially harmful substances, including heavy metals (Expulsia, 2024d).

Choosing the right kind of salt:

Dr. Ray Peat emphasized the significance of using pure white salt without any additives such as iodine and anti-caking agents (Expulsia, 2024d; Ryan Heeney, 2019).

As explained previously too much iodine from supplements or iodinated salt can lead to inflammation of the thyroid gland.

Dr. Ray Peat frequently recommended La Baleine or Morton's canning and pickling salt, both of which are examples of pure white salts without any additives (Expulsia, 2024d).

Natural spices:

It is important to use salt and spices as they enhance the flavor of food, which in turn stimulates the production of digestive enzymes. Natural fresh or dried spices like chili, ginger, garlic, oregano, paprika, and cumin are generally safe. However, be aware that some spices such as pepper can trigger allergic reactions in some people.

Chapter 6: Beverages

Benedicte Mai Lerche MSc PhD

Dangers of Too Much Water

Many people are familiar with the common recommendation to drink eight glasses of water daily, which amounts to about half a gallon or two liters. This guideline often leads individuals to carry a water bottle and diligently try to meet this target (Healthline, 2023)

However, Dr. Ray Peat warned that this advice could be extremely dangerous. He noted that the amount of liquid a person needs varies greatly depending on factors such as metabolic rate, activity level, and environmental conditions like temperature and humidity (Peat R., Water: swelling, tension, pain, fatigue, aging, 2009d).

Dr. Peat also pointed out that forcing oneself to drink a set amount of water daily, regardless of thirst, can trigger harmful adaptive processes. He explained that excessive water consumption has effects similar to those of consuming too little salt. As described in Chapter 6 a low salt diet can create problems with low blood volume, high blood pressure, edema, PMS, and much more (Peat R., Water: swelling, tension, pain, fatigue, aging, 2009d).

When a high water intake is combined with a low-salt diet—which is a common medical recommendation—a healthy individual may adapt easily, but it could have disastrous effects for someone with a slow metabolic rate, as these individuals do not retain salt (sodium) efficiently (Peat R., Water: swelling, tension, pain, fatigue, aging, 2009d).

Dr. Peat emphasized that thirst is the most reliable indicator of your body's liquid needs. He recommended obtaining fluids from milk, tea, coffee, orange juice, and fruits. Unlike pure water, these foods contain minerals and other nutrients that help maintain the body's mineral balance (Peat R., Water: swelling, tension, pain, fatigue, aging, 2009d)

.

Coffee & Tea

Dr. Ray Peat recommended coffee and tea, citing their rich content of nutrients such as caffeine, vitamins, and minerals.

Caffeine boosts the metabolic rate. Caffeine bears notable similarities to thyroid and progesterone, and consuming coffee and tea can help maintain the production of these hormones or compensate for their deficiencies. Additionally, caffeine supports liver function and protects against various degenerative processes (Jodellefit, Dr. Ray Peat on Decaf Coffee, 2020; Peat R., Caffeine: A vitamin-like nutrient, or adaptogen, 2006e).

The health benefits of coffee:

Coffee is a significant source of caffeine and also provides important vitamins and minerals including thiamine (vitamin B1), niacinamide (vitamin B3), magnesium, and manganese (Peat R., Nutrition for Women: 100 Short Articles, 2001d, pp. 75-77).

It is important not to drink black coffee on an empty stomach as caffeine can increase your metabolic rate so much that it depletes the glycogen reserves, leading to a decrease in blood sugar levels. Dr. Ray Peat advised consuming coffee with food or at least adding cream and sugar to your coffee to help stabilize blood sugar and prevent the anxiety-like symptoms that may occur when coffee is consumed alone (Peat R., Caffeine: A vitamin-like nutrient, or adaptogen, 2006e).

The health benefits of tea:

Black tea and green tea contain caffeine, though in lesser amounts compared to coffee. Specifically, coffee has twice the caffeine of black tea and more than three times that of green tea (Hoeffner, 2023). Most herbal teas, such as mint and chamomile, are caffeine-free.

Since teas are derived from leaves, they contain nutrients like magnesium, potassium, and vitamins A, K, E, and Q10, along with B vitamins and other trace minerals, making them nutritionally beneficial (Peat R., Nutrition for Women: 100 Short Articles, 2001d, pp. 75-77).

Since black and green tea contains less caffeine than coffee, there's less concern about combining them with other foods. However, if black tea leads to low blood sugar, causing stress and anxiety, you should combine it with food or add milk and honey to your tea.

Many people avoid drinking coffee late in the evening due to its high caffeine content, which can disrupt sleep. After dinner, opting for an herbal tea can be a good alternative, offering both relaxation and healthy nutrients.

Benedicte Mai Lerche MSc PhD

Alcoholic Drinks

The yeast in alcoholic beverages is estrogenic, and as detailed in Chapter 1, estrogen impairs thyroid function and liver function (Ray Peat Clips, 2016u).

Additionally, the hops in beer are very estrogenic, making beer more estrogenic than other alcoholic drinks (Ray Peat Clips, 2016u).

Dr. Ray Peat noted that beer, wine, and dark-colored liquors such as whiskey, rum, and cognac contain sufficient estrogen to pose a health risk. For a safer alcohol choice, he recommended pure, colorless, highly distilled spirits (Expulsia, 2024b).

Dr. Peat also warned against excessive drinking, as it impairs metabolism and triggers inflammation (Expulsia, 2024b).

Moderate consumption of clear, highly distilled spirits like vodka or gin can offer antioxidant benefits (Expulsia, 2024b). However, some individuals may experience severe allergic reactions to even small amounts of alcohol, exhibiting symptoms like flushing of the face, chest, and sometimes the ears and lips. This could stem from a dramatic hypoglycemic reaction to alcohol, which

Dr. Peat explained can prompt histamine release (Lerche, 2020).

To counteract the blood sugar drop from alcohol, Dr. Peat suggested combining alcohol with fructose. Thus, beverages like vodka mixed with orange juice or cola may be more beneficial (Expulsia, 2024b).

List of Bad & Good Beverages

Bad beverages:

- Drinking too much water when you are not thirsty.
- Black coffee should never be taken on an empty stomach.
- Beer (an occasional beer is okay).
- Wine (wine once in a while is okay).

Good beverages:

Below is a list of healthy beverages. Some of them were presented in the previous chapters under carbohydrates and proteins.

- Coffee (with food or with milk/cream and sugar)
- Tea (black, green, and herbal teas)
- Milk
- Orange juice (without pulp)
- Fruit juices in general
- Lemonades made with natural ingredients
- Cola and other soft drinks (consume in moderation)
- Carbonated water (preferred over still water)
- Colorless, highly distilled spirits (only in small amounts).

Benedicte Mai Lerche MSc PhD

Chapter 7: Food Junk

Benedicte Mai Lerche MSc PhD

Dangerous Additives

Many processed foods, nutritional supplements, and medications can contain harmful additives that may cause issues ranging from allergies to systemic inflammation.

Carrageenan and other thickeners:

Carrageenan, alginate, and agar—all derived from seaweed— microcrystalline cellulose, as well as guar gum, and other gums, are thickeners and emulsifiers commonly used in the food, supplement, and pharmaceutical industries for their gelling, thickening, and stabilizing properties (Peat R., Food-junk and some mystery ailments: Fatigue, Alzheimer's, Colitis, Immunodeficiency., 1995; Functional Performance Systems, 2011a).

Dr. Ray Peat referred to these compounds as novel polymers and explained that they are considered inert materials by the food and drug industry as they are said to be too large to be absorbed through the intestine (Peat R., Food-junk and some mystery ailments: Fatigue, Alzheimer's, Colitis, Immunodeficiency., 1995).

However, Dr. Peat highlighted that these thickeners can dangerously interact with intestinal bacteria and be absorbed directly from the intestine into the bloodstream through a process called "persorption." Once in the bloodstream, they can cause a generalized inflammatory state, potentially leading to degenerative diseases (Peat R., Food-junk and some mystery ailments: Fatigue, Alzheimer's, Colitis, Immunodeficiency., 1995).

Carrageenan is likely the most harmful of the thickeners. It is a powerful allergen and it has been found to cause colitis (inflammation in the colon) as well as anaphylaxis (Functional Performance Systems, 2011a).

It is often present in baby formulas and a wide range of milk products such as ice cream, chocolate milk, frozen yogurt, and cottage cheese. This widespread use has led many to mistakenly believe that milk products are responsible for their allergic symptoms, when in fact, it is the carrageenan causing the reaction (Functional Performance Systems, 2011a).

Carrageenan and other thickeners are also found in many prepared foods including many organic foods.

Binders and fillers in pills:

Nutritional supplements and drugs contain binders and fillers that hold the pill or capsule together. These often include microcrystalline cellulose and small particles such as titanium dioxide and silica (also known as silicon dioxide or colloidal silica). Silica consists of small glass particles (Ray Peat KMUD, 2014).

Dr. Ray Peat expressed significant concern about these compounds. He explained that microcrystalline cellulose is inherently toxic, and the small particles of silica and titanium dioxide can be absorbed from the intestine into the bloodstream, where they activate inflammatory processes (Ray Peat KMUD, 2014).

Sulfites in food and drugs:

Sulfites (sodium bisulfite, potassium metabisulfite, etc.) have long been used as preservatives in foods and drugs, despite their known potential to cause intense allergic reactions in some people, particularly asthmatics (Peat R., Food-junk and some mystery ailments: Fatigue, Alzheimer's, Colitis, Immunodeficiency., 1995). Sulfites are commonly used as preservatives in foods such as dried fruits, preserved meats, pickles, canned vegetables, and wines to prevent darkening and the development of unpleasant odors. They are also commonly used as preservatives in various drugs and medications (Peat R., Food-junk and some mystery ailments: Fatigue, Alzheimer's, Colitis, Immunodeficiency., 1995).

Chapter 8: Pro-Metabolic
Meals

Benedicte Mai Lerche MSc PhD

Combining Foods

In this book, I have outlined Dr. Ray Peat's dietary guidelines. The purpose is to provide you with the knowledge needed to choose fats, carbohydrates, and proteins that support your metabolism. While this book is not a cookbook, this chapter summarizes key points to help you structure your daily eating for optimal results. For meal examples, please visit my website (bochemnordic.com)

Keeping a stable blood sugar:

As discussed throughout this book, maintaining steady blood sugar levels is essential for a high metabolic rate. Low blood sugar directly inhibits the conversion of T4 to the active thyroid hormone T3. Additionally, the stress hormones released in response to low blood sugar decrease the metabolic rate in several ways. Therefore, stabilizing blood sugar is a crucial component of a pro-thyroid diet (Thyroid Patient Advocacy, 2024).

Fasting and going too long without eating can lower blood sugar. It's also important to avoid consuming large amounts of either starch or protein by themselves, as pure glucose (from starch) and pure amino acids from protein will stimulate excessive insulin secretion, resulting in low blood sugar levels. Therefore, it is essential to combine foods correctly to avoid blood sugar disturbances (Peat R., Glycemia, starch, and sugar in context, 2009c).

The importance of complete meals:

By eating fruit (fructose) together with starches and protein, you can prevent their blood sugar-lowering effects. Dr. Ray Peat also suggested preceding a large protein meal with fruits (Ray Peat Clips, 2016o). Additionally, starches are safer when eaten with saturated fats (Functional Performance Systems, 2014; Peat R., From PMS to Menopause: Female Hormones in Context, 2001b, p. 189).

In practice, this means that if you have eggs for breakfast, balancing the egg protein with fruit or orange juice is essential. Starches like potatoes, tortillas, and sourdough bread become less problematic if eaten with fruit and saturated fats.

Whole-balanced meals promote the metabolic rate. By combining good fats, carbohydrates, and proteins from the food list presented in this book, you will be able to create your preferred pro-metabolic meals. Balanced meals also help the body feel satiated and fully nourished, which in turn reduces stress (Peat R., From PMS to Menopause: Female Hormones in Context, 2001b, p. 189).

The ratio of fats, carbohydrates, and proteins in each meal is not critically important as long as you ensure you consume about 100 grams of high-quality protein per day and balance it with a generous amount of fruit or fruit juice (Functional Performance Systems, 2014).

It is important to remember that milk is a balanced meal on its own, containing protein, fats, and sugar. Therefore, dairy products do not need to be balanced with other foods (Peat R., From PMS to Menopause: Female Hormones in Context, 2001b, p. 189).

The importance of frequent eating:

It's crucial not to go too long without eating, as any form of fasting can lower blood sugar and inhibit the production of T3.

Between your main meals, you should have small, balanced snacks. Like your main meals, these snacks should not consist solely of pure protein or pure starch.

Good snack options include fruit, dried fruit (such as raisins), or fruit juice like orange juice. Dairy products, including milk, cheese, Greek yogurt, and homemade ice cream, are also excellent choices. You can also enjoy a cup of homemade cocoa made from milk, cacao powder, and sugar. If you're not very hungry, a cup of tea with milk and honey or sugar can help keep your blood sugar stable.

People prone to hypoglycemia (low blood sugar) should be particularly careful and have many small meals throughout the day. Others who are not hypoglycemic can be less strict.

Combining salt with honey, fruit, or table sugar is especially helpful for stabilizing blood sugar and lowering adrenaline. If you suffer from hypoglycemia or sugar cravings, Dr. Ray Peat advises eating snacks such as salty cheese with sweet fruit (Expulsia, 2011).

Morning blood sugar boost:

When you wake up in the morning, it is important to raise your blood sugar, which has fallen during the night. Dr. Ray Peat emphasized the importance of having something like sweet fruit or orange juice in the morning to bring the blood sugar up. He particularly discouraged exercising on an empty stomach.

Bedtime meal:

Contrary to common advice, Dr. Ray Peat suggested eating before bed.

If you have trouble falling or staying asleep, it might be due to high adrenaline levels. People with a slow metabolism can have adrenaline levels up to 40 times higher than those with good thyroid function.

Trouble falling asleep, staying asleep, and waking up too early often occurs because blood sugar drops, causing an adrenaline spike that can wake you with a pounding heart. According to Dr. Peat, eating a small meal before bedtime can significantly improve sleep by stabilizing blood sugar and preventing the rise of adrenaline.

A good bedtime meal for improving sleep combines salt with fruit, honey, or table sugar. Ideally, a bedtime meal should also include saturated fats and high-quality protein. Examples of good bedtime meals include salty cheese with sweet fruit, homemade ice cream with a little added salt, warm milk with honey together with tortillas with salty cheese (Expulsia, 2011).

Dr. Peat's Weight Loss Tips

You may have initially purchased this book to lose weight, and I trust it has equipped you with the necessary tools to boost your metabolic rate through scientifically supported dietary choices.

However, it's crucial to acknowledge that some individuals who adopt the "Ray Peat diet" may experience weight gain, due to the overconsumption of high-calorie foods like fatty cheese, ice cream, butter, and soft drinks. While these foods are part of the "Ray Peat diet" and can aid in boosting the metabolic rate, they should always be consumed in moderation, especially if you are concerned about your weight or want to lose weight.

In the following, I will outline what a weight-loss version of the "Ray Peat diet" entails.

High-quality protein plays a pivotal role in weight loss by curbing hunger, boosting metabolism, and promoting satiety.

It is extremely important to use plenty of low-fat dairy products, as a high calcium intake helps support metabolism and inhibits fat synthesis.

Opting for low-fat milk and Greek yogurt variants and including cheeses such as mozzarella, feta, and cottage cheese can provide ample calcium and high-quality protein.

Other important sources of protein for weight loss are eggs, shellfish, and gelatin (Strong.Sistas, 2020).

Balancing a protein-rich meal with healthy carbohydrates is essential. Using plenty of sweet low-starch fruits such as pulp-free orange juice, melons, grapes, peaches, etc., will stabilize blood sugar and help promote the production of T3 by your liver (Strong.Sistas, 2020).

It is crucial to limit starch intake – for weight loss, steering clear of bread, pasta, and rice is vital, though well-boiled potatoes eaten with coconut oil and salt remain acceptable.

Coconut oil is more beneficial for weight loss compared to butter. However, it's important to moderate its consumption if you wish to lose weight. Under normal circumstances, around 3 tablespoons of coconut oil per day is fine, but if you have a slow metabolic rate and you want to lose weight, around 1 tablespoons might be more appropriate (Ray Peat Clips, 2016f).

Dr. Ray Peat explained that incorporating his carrot salad or consuming raw carrots alongside a meal can be advantageous for weight loss, as carrots hinder food absorption in the intestine and promote a feeling of fullness, thereby preventing overeating.

In between meals, small snacks of fruit, orange juice, or dairy will help promote the metabolic rate.

It is worth mentioning that gradual, steady weight loss is more sustainable than rapid weight loss. Fast-paced weight loss regimens often entail undereating to a degree that the body perceives as stress, consequently lowering the metabolic rate and making weight loss increasingly challenging. Moreover, once the diet is discontinued, the weight tends to return, often surpassing initial levels, as the metabolic rate has now been reset to a lower level (KUMD, 2013).

It's crucial to highlight that Dr. Ray Peat's dietary principles provide a revolutionary approach to weight loss. Unlike quick fixes, his diet champions a pro-metabolic lifestyle that not only supports weight loss but also enhances overall health and fights aging, inflammation, and disease.

Embracing Dr. Ray Peat's diet principles has been a game-changer for me. I've abandoned traditional dieting entirely. When I want to shed pounds, I confidently follow the weight loss tips outlined above, knowing they are backed by solid scientific research and truly support a healthy, sustainable weight loss journey. This is the only diet out there that genuinely fosters long-term health and well-being while promoting effective weight loss.

Chapter 9: Healing Metabolism

Benedicte Mai Lerche MSc PhD

Balance of Health and Disease

Dr. Ray Peat viewed optimal biological energy production as essential for health and longevity. He argued that stress, inflammation, aging, and disease stem from an imbalance between the body's biological energy resources and environmental demands.

The active thyroid hormone T3 regulates metabolism and thus the conversion of food into biological energy, making thyroid function a key controller of the body's energy resources.

Dr. Peat's health philosophy emphasizes transitioning the body from a low-energy state— marked by low thyroid function (hypothyroidism), stress, and inflammation—to a high-energy state, where abundant cellular energy supports repair and healing.

A crucial first step in Dr. Peat's health philosophy is consistently adopting the dietary principles outlined in this book. For some people, these dietary principles are enough to sufficiently increase the metabolic rate and improve overall health.

However, for others, additional interventions such as thyroid replacement therapy may be necessary.

Dr. Peat has explained that the common practice of relying solely on levothyroxine (T4) to treat hypothyroidism might be inadequate or even problematic, particularly for individuals who have difficulty converting T4 into the active thyroid hormone T3. He advocated for a treatment approach that combines both T4 and T3 in a ratio of about three to one, thereby mimicking the natural secretion of the human thyroid gland.

Additionally, Dr. Peat's health protocol often includes supplementation with the body's natural youth-associated hormones, progesterone and pregnenolone. These hormones are known for their anti-estrogenic, anti-stress, and anti-aging effects. Supplementing these natural hormones can benefit various health issues such as hypothyroidism, stress, inflammation, PMS, infertility, and age-related degenerative conditions.

Dr. Ray Peat's health strategy also includes selected nutritional supplements, probiotics, and light therapy, among others.

It's important to understand that while following Dr. Peat's health principles can lead to swift healing and symptom relief, his philosophy is fundamentally geared towards a long-term commitment to maintaining optimal health and longevity, rather than a quick fix.

For those interested in an introduction to Dr. Peat's health philosophy, my first book, "How I Overcame Hypothyroidism," is an invaluable resource. It details my health journey and the strategies I used to overcome hypothyroidism under Dr. Ray Peat's guidance. This book essentially provides an overview of Dr. Peat's approach to metabolic and hormonal regeneration.

Mastering crucial knowledge about thyroid health and testing is essential for fully healing your metabolism. In my second book, "Test Your Thyroid Function," I explain how you can fall within the so-called normal levels on thyroid lab tests but still be hypothyroid. Drawing on Dr. Ray Peat's expertise, this book empowers you to correctly interpret your thyroid blood test results and use pulse and temperature to track your metabolic rate at home.

This current book is the third installment in the "Healing Metabolism" series. I plan to write additional books, focusing on other aspects of metabolic and hormonal healing inspired by Dr. Ray Peat's research.

Through my website, biochemnordic.com, I offer additional online educational resources that teach you how to implement various aspects of Dr. Ray Peat's pro-metabolic lifestyle, including diet, progesterone, pregnenolone, vitamins and minerals, light therapy, and more. You can also book online video counseling sessions with me through the website.

While visiting biochemnordic.com, you have the option to subscribe to my free mailing list to stay updated on my latest endeavors and other relevant news, including new book publications.

About the Author

Benedicte Mai Lerche earned an MSc in Biochemistry from the University of Copenhagen and a Ph.D. in Chemical and Biochemical Engineering from the Technical University of Denmark.

Benedicte is deeply committed to assisting individuals in overcoming challenges associated with low thyroid function and hormonal imbalances.

Through her website, biochemnordic.com, she provides a wealth of e-learning materials and personalized video counseling, aiming to support individuals worldwide on their health journey.

With a primary focus on supporting optimal thyroid function and boosting cellular energy production, Benedicte shares invaluable knowledge on dietary principles, supplement recommendations, and lifestyle factors that promote efficient metabolism and hormone balance, while also offering anti-aging, anti-stress, and anti-inflammatory benefits.

Driven by the profound impact of Dr. Ray Peat's extensive research, Benedicte has personally witnessed the transformative power of his insights in addressing her own thyroid and hormonal struggles. This experience has fueled her dedication to impart Dr. Peat's invaluable knowledge to others who are encountering similar issues.

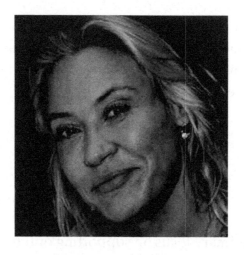

Benedicte Mai Lerche MSc PhD

Your Review Matters

If you found this book valuable, I would be immensely grateful if you could take a moment to leave a review on the platform where you purchased the book or on Goodreads.

Your feedback will help other potential readers facing similar health challenges to discover and benefit from my work.

Just a few thoughtful lines from you can make a significant impact.

Thank you sincerely for your support!

Benedicte Mai Lerche

Benedicte Mai Lerche MSc PhD

References

Linus Pauling Institute. (2024). Fiber - Linus Pauling Institute. *Retrieved from https://lpi.oregonstate.edu/book/export/html/474*

#55: Bioenergetic Nutrition Basics I. (2021). The Ray Peat Diet" I Appetite and Metabolism with Ray Peat. *Retrieved from https://www.youtube.com/watch?v=f06rVi8iXfI*

50k-food health. (2011). Ray Peat Eating Guidelines - Active Low-Carber Forums. *Retrieved from https://50kzone.blogspot.com/2011/06/ray-peat-eating-guidelines-active-low.html*

Alan Jacobs, M. (2023, August 10). What is the Reverse T3 Syndrome? *Retrieved from https://neuroendocrinology.org: https://neuroendocrinology.org/what-is-the-reverse-t3-syndrome/#:~:text=It%20is%20known%20that%20the,this%20as%20the%20RT3%20Syndrome.*

Altınterim, B. (2012). Anti-Thyroid Effects of PUFAS (Polyunsaturated fats) and Herbs. *Retrieved from https://www.researchgate.net/publication/268515453_ANTI-*

THROID_EFFECTS_OF_PUFAS_POLYUNS ATURATED_FATS_AND_HERBS#:~:text=Pol yunsaturated%20fats%20(PUFA)%20suppress %20thyroid,the%20thyroid%20slows%20the%2 0metabolism.

American Society for Biochemistry and Molecular Biology. (2012). Essential Fatty Acids: The Work of George and Mildred Burr. J Biol Chem, *287(42), 35439-35441.*

American Thyroid Association. (2023a). Thyroid Function Tests. *Retrieved August 22, 2023, from https://www.thyroid.org/thyroid-function-tests/*

Another School of Thought Radio. (2011). Dr. Ray Peat: Glycemia, Starch and SUGAR in context! *Retrieved from https://archive.org/details/podcast_another-school-thought-radi_dr-ray-peat-glycemia-starch_1000333787152*

Barnes, B., & Galton, L. (1976). Hypothyroidism The Unsuspected Illness. *HarperCollins.*

BHOF. (2024). A Guide to Calcium-Rich Foods. *Retrieved from https://www.bonehealthandosteoporosis.org/patients/treatment/calciumvitamin-d/a-guide-to-calcium-rich-foods/*

Boston University School of Public Health. (2017). Respiratory health. *Retrieved from https://sphweb.bumc.bu.edu/otlt/MPH-Modules/PH/RespiratoryHealth/*

Brewer, D. T. (2024). Nutrition and Blood Volume Work Together for a Healthy Pregnancy. *Retrieved from http://www.drbrewerpregnancydiet.com/id11.ht ml*

Breyer, M. (2019). 15 Vegetables That Are Actually Fruits. *Retrieved from https://www.treehugger.com/vegetables-are-actually-fruits-4857900*

Britannica. (2024). Meat, fish, and eggs. *Retrieved from https://www.britannica.com/science/human-nutrition/Meat-fish-and-eggs*

Centra food. (2024). Centra Food. *Retrieved from https://www.centrafoods.com/products/oils-list*

Cleveland Clinic. (2019). Thyroid Issues? What You Should Know About Foods and Supplements to Avoid. *Retrieved from https://health.clevelandclinic.org/thyroid-issues-what-you-need-to-know-about-diet-and-supplements/*

Cleveland Clinic. (2021). Parathyroid Hormone. *Retrieved   from https://my.clevelandclinic.org/health/articles/223 55-parathyroid-hormone*

Cleveland Clinic. (2022c). Collagen. *Retrieved from https://my.clevelandclinic.org/health/articles/230 89-collagen*

Diet Doctor. (2024b). Plant protein vs. animal protein: Which one is healthier for you? *Retrieved from https://www.dietdoctor.com/high-protein/plant-vs-animal-protein*

Doctor, Diet. (2024a). Vegetable oils: Are they healthy? *Retrieved   from https://www.dietdoctor.com/low-carb/vegetable-oils*

Dynamic Science. (2024). Lesson 3 Rancidity. *Retrieved   from http://www.dynamicscience.com.au/tester/soluti ons1/chemistry/organic/Lesson3%20ranciditysol n.pdf*

Eluv Radio 2014 Stress and Trauma. (2014b). Ray Peat on livers nutritional value. *Retrieved from https://www.youtube.com/watch?v=7mVXtXP W_D0*

Eluv Radio: Stress and Trauma. (2014a). Ray Peat on eating a vegetarian diet. *Retrieved from*

https://www.youtube.com/watch?v=BnBF7xOW
Wew

Eluv Radio: Stress and Trauma. (2014c). Ray Peat on eating a daily carrot. *Retrieved from https://www.youtube.com/watch?v=wfnH0lc2Bl s*

Enviromedica. (2024). Beef Liver: Nature's Perfect Food. *Retrieved from https://enviromedica.com/blogs/learn/beef-liver-natures-perfect-food#:~:text=Liver%20is%20an%20excellent%20source,D%2C%20E%2C%20K).*

Erlanson-Albertsson C, S. K. (2021). The Importance of Food for Endotoxemia and an Inflammatory Response. International Journal of Molecular Sciences, 22(17). *Retrieved from https://www.ncbi.nlm.nih.gov/pmc/articles/PMC8431640/*

Everyday Health. (2018). Do You Really Need to Give Up Kale, Cauliflower, and Other Cruciferous Vegetables When You Have Hypothyroidism? *Retrieved from https://www.everydayhealth.com/hs/hypothyroidism/do-you-need-to-avoid-cruciferous-vegetables/*

Expulsia. (2011). East West: Glycemia, Starch and Sugar in context. *Retrieved from https://www.toxinless.com/ewh-110427-glycemia-starch-and-sugar-in-context.mp3*

Expulsia. (2024a). Ray Peat E-mail Exchange: Gelatin. *Retrieved from https://expulsia.com/health/emailexchanges#Gelatin*

Expulsia. (2024b). Ray Peat E-mail exchange: Alcohol. *Retrieved from https://expulsia.com/health/emailexchanges#Alcohol*

Expulsia. (2024c). Ray Peat E-mail exchange: Sourdough bread. *Retrieved from https://expulsia.com/health/emailexchanges#Sourdough_bread*

Expulsia. (2024d). Ray Peat Email Exchanges: Salt. *Retrieved from https://expulsia.com/health/emailexchanges#Salt*

Farag MA, G. M. (2022). Omega-9 fatty acids: potential roles in inflammation and cancer management. J Genet Eng Biotechnol., 1(48).

Food Research International. (2021). Potato protein: An emerging source of high quality and allergy free protein, and its possible future based products. *Retrieved from https://www.sciencedirect.com/science/article/abs/pii/S0963996921004828*

Functional Performance. (2012). Ray Peat, PhD on Endotoxin. *Retrieved from https://www.functionalps.com/blog/2012/11/29/ray-peat-phd-on-endotoxin/*

Functional Performance Systems. (2011a). Carrageenan, Inflammation, Cancer, Immunity. *Retrieved from https://www.functionalps.com/blog/2011/11/11/carrageenan-inflammation-cancer-immunity/*

Functional Performance Systems. (2011b). Dairy, Calcium, and Weight Management in Adults and Children. *Retrieved from https://www.functionalps.com/blog/2011/11/02/milk-calcium-and-weight-loss-in-adults-and-children/*

Functional Performance Systems. (2012a). Toxicity of Stored PUFA. *Retrieved from https://www.functionalps.com/blog/2012/04/22/fatty-acid-composition-of-diet-reflected-in-fat-tissue/*

Functional performance Systems. (2012b). Ray Peat, PhD Quotes on Coconut Oil. *Retrieved from https://www.functionalps.com/blog/2012/03/19/ray-peat-phd-on-coconut-oil/*

Functional Performance Systems. (2014). Ray Peat, PhD – Concerns with Starches. *Retrieved from*

*https://www.functionalps.com/blog/2014/06/06/r
ay-peat-phd-concerns-with-starches/*

Functional Performance Systems. (2024a). Ray Peat,
PhD on Low Blood Sugar & Stress Reaction.
*Retrieved   from
https://www.functionalps.com/blog/2012/11/26/r
ay-peat-phd-on-low-blood-sugar-stress-reaction/*

Functional Performance Systems. (2024b). Ray Peat,
PhD on the Benefits of the Raw Carrot.
*Retrieved   from
https://www.functionalps.com/blog/2012/09/28/r
ay-peat-phd-on-the-benefits-of-the-raw-carrot/*

George F Cahill Jr, R. L. (2003). Ketoacids? Good
medicine?   *Retrieved   from
https://pubmed.ncbi.nlm.nih.gov/12813917/*

Get Cracking. (2023). Here's Why Your Omega-3
Eggs May Smell Fishy. *Retrieved from
https://www.getcracking.ca/recipes/article/heres-
why-your-omega-3-eggs-may-smell-fishy*

Glanbia Nutritionals. (2024). Glanbia Nutritionals.
*Retrieved   from
https://www.glanbianutritionals.com/en/nutri-
knowledge-center/nutritional-resources/what-
are-
mcts#:~:text=In%20general%2C%20when%20*

working%20with,point%20than%20long%20ch
ain%20triglycerides.*

Great Lakes Wellness. (2014). Great Lakes Wellness.
Retrieved from https://greatlakeswellness.com/

Harvard Medical School. (2022). The truth about fats:
the good, the bad, and the in-between.
*Retrieved   from
https://www.health.harvard.edu/staying-
healthy/the-truth-about-fats-bad-and-
good#:~:text=A%20polyunsaturated%20fat%20
has%20two,Both%20types%20offer%20health%
20benefits.*

Harvard T.H. Chan. (2024). Carbohydrates and Blood
Sugar. *Retrieved   from
https://www.hsph.harvard.edu/nutritionsource/c
arbohydrates/carbohydrates-and-blood-sugar/*

Harward T. H. Chan . (2024). Whole Grains. *Retrieved
from
https://www.hsph.harvard.edu/nutritionsource/
what-should-you-eat/whole-grains/*

Health Line. (2023). Omega-3-6-9 Fatty Acids: A
Complete Overview. *Retrieved from
https://www.healthline.com/nutrition/omega-3-
6-9-overview#food-sources*

Health Line. (2023). Top 13 Lean Protein Foods.
Retrieved   from

https://www.healthline.com/nutrition/lean-
protein-foods#fish

Healthbeet.org. (2024). High Protein. *Retrieved from*
https://healthbeet.org/wp-
content/uploads/2020/09/high-protien-list-of-
foods-with-calories-and-grams-of-protein.pdf

HealthLine. (2022). 9 Health Benefits of Eating Eggs.
Retrieved   from
https://www.healthline.com/nutrition/proven-
health-benefits-of-eggs

Healthline. (2023). Drink 8 Glasses of Water a Day:
Fact   or   Fiction?   *Retrieved   from*
https://www.healthline.com/nutrition/8-glasses-
of-water-per-day#TOC_TITLE_HDR_2

Healthline. (2023). Glycemic Index: What It Is and
How   to   Use   It.   *Retrieved   from*
https://www.healthline.com/nutrition/glycemic-
index

Healthline. (2023). Refined vs. Unrefined Coconut
Oil: What's the Difference? *Retrieved from*
https://www.healthline.com/nutrition/refined-vs-
unrefined-coconut-oil#production

Henrik Parbo, A. N. (2015). Fedtstoffer. In Kend
Kemien 1 *(pp. 202- 2016). Gyldendal.*

Herb Doctors. (2018). Herb Doctors: Milk. *Retrieved*
from

https://www.youtube.com/watch?v=41POVqM WEIg

Hoeffner, M. K. (2023). Coffee vs. Tea: Which One Is Better for You? *Retrieved from https://www.realsimple.com/coffee-or-tea-7253639*

International Osteoporosis Foundation. (2024). Calcium content of common foods. *Retrieved from https://www.osteoporosis.foundation/calcium-content-of-common-foods*

Iowa State University Extension and Outreach. (2019). VEGETABLE OILS – COMPARISON, COST, AND NUTRITION. *Retrieved from https://spendsmart.extension.iastate.edu/spends mart/2013/08/19/vegetable-oils-comparison-cost-and-nutrition/*

Jodellefit. (2020). Dr. Ray Peat - Iodine, Spider Veins, Oxalates, Fat Loss, & More Listener questions answered! *Retrieved from https://www.youtube.com/watch?v=6uTJLfQUJ Os&t=2202s*

Jodellefit. (2020). Dr. Ray Peat on Decaf Coffee. *Retrieved from https://www.youtube.com/watch?v=drUqU4cKo EA*

Jodellefit. (2021). Dr. Ray Peat - Liver Health, Milk, Alcohol, and More Listener Q&A. *Retrieved from* *https://www.youtube.com/watch?v=CTvB9lDk5 PM*

Johns Hopkins medicine. (2024). PROTEIN CONTENT OF COMMON FOODS. *Retrieved from https://www.hopkinsmedicine.org/-/media/bariatrics/nutrition_protein_content_co mmon_foods.pdf*

Jorge L. Rosado, 1. M. (2005). Calcium Absorption from Corn Tortilla Is Relatively High and Is Dependent upon Calcium Content and Liming in Mexican Women. The Journal Of Nutrtion , *135(11), 2578-2581. Retrieved from https://jn.nutrition.org/content/135/11/2578.lon g*

Kaur N, C. V. (2014). Essential fatty acids as functional components of foods- a review. J Food Sci Technol., 51(10), 2289-303.

Khan Academy. (2024). Gluconeogenesis: the big picture. *Retrieved from https://www.khanacademy.org/test-prep/mcat/biomolecules/carbohydrate-metabolism/v/gluconeogenesis*

Khan Academy. (2024). Lipids. *Retrieved from https://www.khanacademy.org/science/biology/m acromolecules/lipids/a/lipids*

KMUD. (2011). Sodium, Salt, Inflammation, Pregnancy Toxeamia, Water Retention. *Retrieved from https://www.youtube.com/watch?v=zwmDaU4z Q8o&t=1393s*

KMUD. (2012). Ray Peat on general dietary advice on preventing blocked arteries. *Retrieved from https://www.youtube.com/watch?v=-dLzXyVi4Xw*

KMUD. (2012). Ray Peat on salt, blood sugar, adrenaline. *Retrieved from https://www.youtube.com/watch?v=QS2lM6tkT 1U*

KMUD. (2015). Digestion and Emotion Full Interview. *Retrieved from https://www.youtube.com/watch?v=vr9rktGm1 Mg*

KMUD: Blood Pressure Regulation Heart Failure and Muscle Atrophy . (2012). Ray Peat on salt, blood sugar, adrenaline. *Retrieved from https://www.youtube.com/watch?v=QS2lM6tkT 1U*

KMUD: Bowel Endotoxin. (2009). Ray Peat on ways to improve endotoxin, aspirin, laxatives, carrot, bamboo. *Retrieved from https://www.youtube.com/watch?v=-6GuqunKdPQ*

KMUD: Food. (2016). Ray Peat on what he normally eats. *Retrieved from https://www.youtube.com/watch?v=iSlgnvswjdU*

Koshland, D. E. (2014). Protein. *Retrieved from https://www.britannica.com/science/protein*

KUMD. (2013). Ray Peat on calories, stress, when a pure fat diet would work. Muscles. Weight loss. *Retrieved from https://www.youtube.com/watch?v=feAV58jgALs*

Lam, K. (2022). The Difference Between Pastured, Organic, and Free Range Eggs. *Retrieved from https://delishably.com/dairy/How-to-buy-the-healthiest-eggs*

Lerche, B. M. (2020, December 3). Email excahnge with DR. Ray Peat.

Linus Pauling Institute. (2024). Essential Fatty Acids. *Retrieved from https://lpi.oregonstate.edu/mic/other-nutrients/essential-fatty-acids#introduction*

Mamounis, K. J. (2017). The Dangers of Fat Metabolism and PUFA: Why You Don't Want to be a Fat Burner. Journal of Evolution and Health, 2(1).

Mary Shomon. (2022). Overview of Reverse T3 Thyroid Hormone. *Retrieved from https://www.verywellhealth.com/reverse-t3-thyroid-hormone-overview-3233184#toc-possible-significance*

Medical News Today. (2018). What are phytoestrogens? Benefits and foods. *Retrieved from https://www.medicalnewstoday.com/articles/320630*

Medical News Today. (2023a). Top 15 sources of plant-based protein. *Retrieved from https://www.medicalnewstoday.com/articles/321474*

Medical News Today. (2023b). What to know about eating legumes. *Retrieved from https://www.medicalnewstoday.com/articles/what-are-legumes#drawbacks*

Medical News Today. (2024). What to know about sugar in fruit. *Retrieved from https://www.medicalnewstoday.com/articles/325550#potential-risks*

Medline Plus. (2024). Blood Glucose. *Retrieved from https://medlineplus.gov/bloodglucose.html#:~:tex t=Blood%20glucose%2C%20or%20blood%20su gar,your%20pancreas%20to%20release%20insu lin.*

Nashoba Brook Bakery Bread . (2024). gluten-sensitivity. *Retrieved from https://slowrise.com/gluten-sensitivity*

National Council on Strength and Fitness. (2024). EARLY MORNING WORKOUT: TO EAT OR NOT TO EAT? *Retrieved from https://www.ncsf.org/blog/163-early-morning-workout-to-eat-or-not-to-eat*

Nava, A. S., & Raja., A. (2022). Physiology, Metabolism. National Library of Medicine, 12.

OnePeak Medical. (2024). Collagen vs Gelatin: What's the Difference? *Retrieved from https://www.onepeakmedical.com/collagen-vs-gelatin/*

Open Biotechnology Journal. (2019). Antinutrients in Plant-based Foods: A Review. *Retrieved from https://openbiotechnologyjournal.com/VOLUME /13/PAGE/68/FULLTEXT/*

Open Oregon. (2020b). Introduction to Carbohydrates. *Retrieved from https://openoregon.pressbooks.pub/nutritionscien ce/chapter/unit-4-introduction-carbohydrates/*

Open Oregon. (2020c). Digestion and Absorption of Carbohydrates. *Retrieved from https://openoregon.pressbooks.pub/nutritionscien ce/chapter/4c-digestion-absorption-carbohydrates/*

Open Oregon. (2020d). Types of Carbohydrates. *Retrieved from https://openoregon.pressbooks.pub/nutritionscien ce/chapter/4a-types-of-carbohydrates/*

Open Oregon. (2020e). Glucose Regulation and Utilization in the Body. *Retrieved from https://openoregon.pressbooks.pub/nutritionscien ce/chapter/4d-glucose-regulation-utilization-body/*

Open Oregon. (2020f). Fatty Acid Types and Food Sources. *Retrieved from https://openoregon.pressbooks.pub/nutritionscien ce/chapter/5c-fatty-acid-types-food-sources/*

Open Oregon. (2020g). Lipid Types and Structures. *Retrieved from https://openoregon.pressbooks.pub/nutritionscien ce/chapter/5b-lipid-types-structures/*

Open Oregon Educational Science. (2020a). Protein Structure. *Retrieved from https://openoregon.pressbooks.pub/nutritionscien ce/chapter/6a-protein-structure/*

Peat, R. (1995). Food-junk and some mystery ailments: Fatigue, Alzheimer's, Colitis, Immunodeficiency. *(https://raypeat.com/articles/nutrition/carrageen an.shtml ed.).*

Peat, R. (2001a). Generative Energy: Restoring the Wholeness of Life. *Raymond Peat PhD.*

Peat, R. (2001b). From PMS to Menopause: Female Hormones in Context. *Raymond Peat Ph.D.*

Peat, R. (2001c). Progesterone in Orthomolecular Medicine. *Raymond Peat Phd.*

Peat, R. (2001d). Nutrition for Women: 100 Short Articles. *Raymond Peat Ph.D.*

Peat, R. (2004, January). Gelatin, stress, longevity. Ray Peat's newsletter, *1-8.*

Peat, R. (2006a). Unsaturated Vegetable Oils: Toxic. *Retrieved from https://raypeat.com/articles/articles/unsaturated-oils.shtml*

Peat, R. (2006b). Coconut Oil. *Retrieved from https://raypeat.com/articles/articles/coconut-oil.shtml*

Peat, R. (2006c). Vegetables, etc.—Who Defines Food? *Retrieved from https://raypeat.com/articles/articles/vegetables.sh tml*

Peat, R. (2006d). Tryptophan, serotonin, and aging. *Retrieved from https://raypeat.com/articles/aging/tryptophan-serotonin-aging.shtml*

Peat, R. (2006e). Caffeine: A vitamin-like nutrient, or adaptogen. *Retrieved from https://raypeat.com/articles/articles/caffeine.shtm l*

Peat, R. (2006f). Iron's Dangers. *Retrieved from https://raypeat.com/articles/articles/iron-dangers.shtml*

Peat, R. (2007a). Cholesterol, longevity, intelligence, and health. *Retrieved from https://raypeat.com/articles/articles/cholesterol-longevity.shtml*

Peat, R. (2007b). Unsaturated fatty acids: Nutritionally essential, or toxic? *Retrieved from https://raypeat.com/articles/articles/unsaturatedf ats.shtml*

Peat, R. (2007c). The Great Fish Oil Experiment. *Retrieved from https://raypeat.com/articles/articles/fishoil.shtml*

Peat, R. (2008a, January). TSH, temperature, pulse rate, and other indicators in hypothyroidism. Ray Peat's Newsletter, 2-6.

Peat, R. (2008b). Natural estrogens. *Retrieved from https://raypeat.com/articles/articles/natural-estrogens.shtml*

Peat, R. (2009a). Fats and degeneration. *Retrieved from https://raypeat.com/articles/articles/fats-degeneration3.shtml*

Peat, R. (2009b). Calcium and Disease: Hypertension, organ calcification, & shock, vs. respiratory energy. *Retrieved from https://raypeat.com/articles/articles/calcium.shtml*

Peat, R. (2009c). Glycemia, starch, and sugar in context. *Retrieved from https://raypeat.com/articles/articles/glycemia.shtml*

Peat, R. (2009d). Water: swelling, tension, pain, fatigue, aging. *Retrieved from https://raypeat.com/articles/articles/water.shtml*

Peat, R. (2011). Milk in context: allergies, ecology, and some myths. *Retrieved from* *https://raypeat.com/articles/articles/milk.shtml*

Peat, R. (2013). Fats, functions & malfunctions. *Retrieved from* *https://raypeat.com/articles/articles/fats-functions-malfunctions.shtml*

Peat, R. (2015). Mushrooms-observations and interpretations. Ray Peat's Newsletter, *pp. 1-7.*

Peat, R. (2016a). Glucose and sucrose for diabetes. *Retrieved from* *https://raypeat.com/articles/articles/glucose-sucrose-diabetes.shtml*

Peat, R. (2016b). Salt, energy, metabolic rate, and longevity. *Retrieved from* *https://raypeat.com/articles/articles/salt.shtml*

Peat, R. (2017). Ray Peat Eluv Radio 2014 Stress and Trauma. *Retrieved from* *https://www.youtube.com/watch?v=dEd-OmoHszg*

Ravnskov U, D. D. (2016). Lack of an association or an inverse association between low-density-lipoprotein cholesterol and mortality in the elderly: a systematic review. BMJ Open., *12;6((6):e010401).*

Ravnskov U, d. L. (2018). LDL-C does not cause cardiovascular disease: a comprehensive review of the current literature. Expert Rev Clin Pharmacol., 11(10), 959-970.

Ravnskov, U. (2020). DET "ONDE" KOLESTEROL ER VORES BEDSTE VEN. *Retrieved from https://www.dsom.dk/wp-content/uploads/2020/01/Det-22onde22-kolesterol-er-vores-bedste-ven-Uffe-Ravnskov-1.pdf*

Ray Peat. (2013). Phosphate, activation, and aging. *Retrieved from https://raypeat.com/articles/articles/phosphate-activation-aging.shtml*

Ray Peat clips. (2009). Ray Peat on leaky gut and causes of it. *Retrieved from https://www.youtube.com/watch?v=6zASL2i5brM*

Ray Peat Clips. (2010a). Ray Peat on amino acid requirements, methionine and life span. *Retrieved from https://www.youtube.com/watch?v=rVZATrhJ02Q*

Ray Peat Clips. (2010b). Ray Peat on chicken eggs. #2. *Retrieved from https://www.youtube.com/watch?v=rxgt2JkXzd M*

Ray Peat Clips. (2010c). Ray Peat KMUD: 9-17-10 Sugar part 1 Full Interview. *Retrieved from https://www.youtube.com/watch?v=Lx96YYKv A9w*

Ray Peat Clips. (2014a). Ray Peat on carotene in sweet potatoes #2. *Retrieved from https://www.youtube.com/watch?v=vCOpp8qRl _Q*

Ray Peat clips. (2014b). Ray Peat on potato juice fixing ammonia problems, assimilating protein. *Retrieved from https://www.youtube.com/watch?v=PaiL_Z_e03 I*

Ray Peat Clips. (2016a). Ray Peat on thyroid labs and T3, T4, rT3, TSH. *Retrieved August 10, 2023, from https://www.youtube.com/watch?v=HynVEuBi CpM*

Ray Peat Clips. (2016b). Ray Peat on the Burr's fat free diet research, EFA deficiency, nutritional deficiencies. *Retrieved from https://www.youtube.com/watch?v=Oc1ijSN220 k&t=13s*

Ray Peat Clips. (2016d). Ray Peat on MCT oils. *Retrieved   from* *https://www.youtube.com/watch?v=SGFbTnfUv NI*

Ray Peat Clips. (2016e). Ray Peat on the importance of the liver and liver health. *Retrieved from https://www.youtube.com/watch?v=wxTwBY5r _qA*

Ray Peat Clips. (2016f). Ray Peat on storing PUFA. *Retrieved   from* *https://www.youtube.com/watch?v=559VNn-Z924*

Ray Peat Clips. (2016g). Ray Peat on the best meat to eat. *Retrieved   from* *https://www.youtube.com/watch?v=-dLzXyVi4Xw*

Ray Peat Clips. (2016h). Ray Peat on general protein requirements. *Retrieved   from* *https://www.youtube.com/watch?v=Ygyxqxlx51 U*

Ray Peat Clips. (2016i). Ray Peat on Lactic acid foods and metabolism and migranes. *Retrieved from https://www.youtube.com/watch?v=581jh9sv3n 0*

Ray Peat Clips. (2016j). Ray Peat on how many potatoes needed to get enough protein.

Retrieved from
https://www.youtube.com/watch?v=Vd8lIEfF_t4

Ray Peat Clips. (2016k). Ray Peat on yoghurt, best type of yoghurt to eat and kefir lactic acid. *Retrieved from https://www.youtube.com/watch?v=8ErddLqGZ M4*

Ray Peat Clips. (2016l). Ray Peat on food choices and endotoxin. *Retrieved from https://www.youtube.com/watch?v=oK5zPpc_m y0*

Ray Peat Clips. (2016m). Ray Peat on best type of fiber. *Retrieved from https://www.youtube.com/watch?v=TPVPdv3Yf EA*

Ray Peat Clips. (2016n). Ray Peat on the benefits of fructose. *Retrieved from https://www.youtube.com/watch?v=uXuuPqPX rOw*

Ray Peat Clips. (2016o). Ray Peat on different types of starch, food combinations, whole grains, legumes, beans. *Retrieved from https://www.youtube.com/watch?v=aAkcGGoF Me0*

Ray Peat Clips. (2016ø). Ray Peat on saturated fat protecting against endotoxin. Eating fat with starch. *Retrieved from https://www.youtube.com/watch?v=-XNN236xGwM*

Ray Peat Clips. (2016p). Ray Peat on the "good and bad bacteria" idea in the gut. *Retrieved from https://www.youtube.com/watch?v=fsrUZvk7Cj E*

Ray Peat clips. (2016q). Ray Peat on the effects of diet devoid of sugar and general diet advice. *Retrieved from https://www.youtube.com/watch?v=jQw1SJ3UF ww*

Ray Peat Clips. (2016r). Ray Peat on glycogen storage and depletion. *Retrieved from https://www.youtube.com/watch?v=ZV468c8ljn c*

Ray Peat Clips. (2016s). Ray Peat on benefits of fructose #2 insulin. *Retrieved from https://www.youtube.com/watch?v=nlG8vV2hD g8*

Ray Peat clips. (2016t). Ray Peat on poorly digested starch's effects, endotoxin, fat gain, insulin. *Retrieved from https://www.youtube.com/watch?v=S2KAGuStt CI*

Ray Peat Clips. (2016u). Ray Peat on alcoholic drinks. *Retrieved from* https://www.youtube.com/watch?v=wwaGrhK66 H4

Ray Peat Clips. (2016v). Ray Peat on how to minimize starch negatives. *Retrieved from* https://www.youtube.com/watch?v=4Vtxh5D5p ds

Ray Peat Clips. (2016x). Ray Peat on eating a healthy vegan diet. *Retrieved from* https://www.youtube.com/watch?v=7hzgt0wGul A

Ray Peat Clips. (2016y). Ray Peat on the harmful effects of endotoxin, hormonal changes. *Retrieved from* https://www.youtube.com/watch?v=YicUmuJVr sQ

Ray Peat Clips. (2016z). Ray Peat on carotene, infertility. *Retrieved from* https://www.youtube.com/watch?v=z76fzyHwhq M

Ray Peat clips. (2017). Ray Peat on carotene in sweet potatoes and the effects on thyroid. *Retrieved from* https://www.youtube.com/watch?v=7WUd_Spv QTY

Ray Peat Clips. (2017b). Ray Peat on saturated fat protecting against stored unsaturated fats. Coconut oil with meals. *Retrieved from https://www.youtube.com/watch?v=1mdwKp4sn cc*

Ray Peat Clips. (2023). Raw Liver & Eggs (Ray Peat). *Retrieved from https://www.youtube.com/watch?v=bRSMT8pw gkQ*

Ray Peat Clips KMUD. (2016c). Ray Peat on reasonable daily calcium intake, calcium supplements. *Retrieved from https://www.youtube.com/watch?v=yl2JdcXrVh E*

Ray Peat KMUD. (2008). Thyroid and Polyunsaturated Fatty Acids Full Interview. *Retrieved from https://www.youtube.com/watch?v=kBhuoW8z QFo*

Ray Peat KMUD. (2014). Ray Peat on modified cellulose, silica, additives in supplements. *Retrieved from https://www.youtube.com/watch?v=DkwvGn33 1pQ*

Ray Peat KMUD Food Additives Full Interview. (2009g). Ray Peat KMUD Food Additives Full

Interview. *Retrieved from https://www.youtube.com/watch?v=uxdLc6sntsQ*

Reid-McCann RJ, B. S. (2022). *The effect of animal versus plant protein on muscle mass, muscle strength, physical performance and sarcopenia in adults: protocol for a systematic review.* Systematic review, 11(1).

Roddy, D. (2016). Safe Supplements with Ray Peat [Generative Energy #31]. *Retrieved from https://www.youtube.com/watch?v=PuSfV43Quuo*

Rogers, K. (2016). What Is the Difference Between a Peptide and a Protein? Encyclopedia Britannica. *Retrieved from https://www.britannica.com/story/what-is-the-difference-between-a-peptide-and-a-protein*

Rogers, K. (2024). Goitrogen. *Retrieved from https://www.britannica.com/science/dietary-supplement*

Rosch, P. J. (2008). *Cholesterol does not cause coronary heart disease in contrast to stress.* Scandinavian Cardiovascular Journal, 42(4), 244-249.

Ryan Heeney. (2018). Dr. Ray Peat on Cortisol and Ketogenic/Low Carbohydrate Diets.

Retrieved *from*
https://www.youtube.com/watch?v=dLet4146j08

Ryan Heeney. (2019). Ray Peat on Iodine. *Retrieved from*
https://www.youtube.com/watch?v=VA5D4qzge js

Saini RK, P. P. (2021). Omega–3 Polyunsaturated Fatty Acids (PUFAs): Emerging Plant and Microbial Sources, Oxidative Stability, Bioavailability, and Health Benefits—A Review. Antioxidants (Basel), 10(10), 1627.

Saventes. (2022). Fatty Acid Ratios. *Retrieved from*
https://savantes.org/news-and-articles/cooking-and-using-olive-oil/72-fatty-acid-ratios#:~:text=Olive%20oil%20has%2070%2D80,high%20level%20of%20saturated%20fats

Society of Endocrinology. (2020, January). Thyroid Gland. *Retrieved from You and Your hormones:*
https://www.yourhormones.info/glands/thyroid-gland/

Sokoła-Wysoczańska, E. W.-S. (2018). Polyunsaturated Fatty Acids and Their Potential Therapeutic Role in Cardiovascular System Disorders—A Review. Nutrients, 10(10), 1561. *Retrieved from*
https://www.ncbi.nlm.nih.gov/pmc/articles/PMC6213446/#:~:text=Omega%20fatty%20acids%

20are%20classified,3%20and%20omega%2D6
%20families.

Speakman, J. (2024). Mind & Matter Podcast .
Retrieved from
https://www.youtube.com/watch?v=KEZFpXUa
8H0

Strong.Sistas. (2020). Dr Ray Peat Q&A | PUFAS,
fructose, weight loss, PCOS, hormones,
cholesterol, & more. *Retrieved from*
https://www.youtube.com/watch?v=96AFY50-
J4A

Study Mind. (2024). Lipids and Triglycerides (A-
level Biology). *Retrieved February 2024, from*
https://studymind.co.uk/notes/lipids-and-
triglycerides/

The American Journal of Clinical Nutrition. (1980). A
mathematical relationship between the fatty
acid composition of the diet and that of the
adipose tissue in man. *Retrieved from*
https://ajcn.nutrition.org/article/S0002-
9165(23)43753-7/abstract

Thyroid Patient Advocacy. (2024). An Interview With
Dr. Raymond Peat who offers his thoughts
about Thyroid Disease. *Retrieved from*
https://www.tpauk.com/main/article/an-

interview-with-dr-raymond-peat-who-offers-his-thoughts-about-thyroid-disease/

US Department of Agriculture. (2018). Gelatins, dry powder, unsweetened. *Retrieved from https://fdc.nal.usda.gov/fdc-app.html#/food-details/169599/nutrients*

Vander, A. J., Sherman, J. H., & Luciano, D. S. (2001). Human Physiology: The Mechanisms of Body Function. *McGraw-Hill.*

Very Well Fit. (2022). Beef Liver Nutrition Facts and Health Benefits. *Retrieved from https://www.verywellfit.com/beef-liver-nutrition-facts-and-health-benefits-5025125*

Web MD. (2023). Is Eating Liver Good for You? Benefits and Risks. *Retrieved from https://www.webmd.com/diet/liver-good-for-you*

Wilson, D. (2015, June). Low Body Temperature as an Indicator for Poor Expression of Thyroid Hormone. (C. Gustafson, Ed.) Integrative Medicine, 14(3), 24–28.

Visit
BiochemNordic.com

Made in the USA
Las Vegas, NV
21 January 2025

16742431R00174